Cancer Emergencies

Guest Editors

MOHAMUD DAYA, MD, MS
DAVID M. SPIRO, MD, MPH
CHARLES R. THOMAS Jr, MD

HEMATOLOGY/ONCOLOGY CLINICS OF NORTH AMERICA

www.hemonc.theclinics.com

Consulting Editors
GEORGE P. CANELLOS, MD
NANCY BERLINER, MD

June 2010 • Volume 24 • Number 3

SAUNDERS an imprint of ELSEVIER, Inc.

W.B. SAUNDERS COMPANY
A Division of Elsevier Inc.

1600 John F. Kennedy Blvd. • Suite 1800 • Philadelphia, PA 19103-2899

http://www.theclinics.com

HEMATOLOGY/ONCOLOGY CLINICS OF NORTH AMERICA Volume 24, Number 3
June 2010 ISSN 0889-8588, ISBN 13: 978-1-4377-2528-5

Editor: Kerry Holland

Hematology/Oncology Clinics (ISSN 0889-8588) is published bimonthly by Elsevier Inc., 360 Park Avenue South, New York, NY 10010-1710. Months of issue are February, April, June, August, October, and December. Business and Editorial Offices: 1600 John F. Kennedy Blvd., Ste. 1800, Philadelphia, PA 19103–2899. Customer Service Office: 3251 Riverport Lane, Maryland Heights, MO 63043. Periodicals postage paid at New York, NY and at additional mailing offices. Subscription prices are $306.00 per year (domestic individuals), $483.00 per year (domestic institutions), $152.00 per year (domestic students/residents), $347.00 per year (Canadian individuals), $591.00 per year (Canadian institutions) $413.00 per year (international individuals), $591.00 per year (international institutions), and $206.00 per year (international and Canadian students/residents). International air speed delivery is included in all *Clinics* subscription prices. All prices are subject to change without notice. **POSTMASTER:** Send address changes to *Hematology/Oncology Clinics of North America*, Elsevier Health Sciences Division, Subscription Customer Service, 3251 Riverport Lane, Maryland Heights, MO 63043. Customer Service (orders, claims, online, change of address): Elsevier Health Sciences Division, Subscription Customer Service, 3251 Riverport Lane, Maryland Heights, MO 63043. Tel: 1-800-654-2452 (U.S. and Canada); 314-447-8871 (outside U.S. and Canada). Fax: 314-447-8029. E-mail: journalscustomerservice-usa@elsevier.com (for print support); journalsonlinesupport-usa@elsevier.com (for online support).

Reprints. For copies of 100 or more, of articles in this publication, please contact the Commercial Reprints Department, Elsevier Inc., 360 Park Avenue South, New York, New York 10010-1710; Tel.: 212-633-3813, Fax: 212-462-1935, E-mail: reprints@elsevier.com.

Hematology/Oncology Clinics of North America is covered in *MEDLINE/PubMed (Index Medicus), EMBASE/Excerpta Medica,* and *BIOSIS.*

Printed and bound by CPI Group (UK) Ltd, Croydon, CR0 4YY

Transferred to Digital Print 2011

Contributors

CONSULTING EDITORS

GEORGE P. CANELLOS, MD
William Rosenberg Professor of Medicine, Department of Medical Oncology,
Dana-Farber Cancer Institute, Boston, Massachusetts

NANCY BERLINER, MD
Chief, Division of Hematology, Brigham and Women's Hospital; Professor of Medicine,
Harvard Medical School, Boston, Massachusetts

GUEST EDITORS

MOHAMUD DAYA, MD, MS
Associate Professor, Department of Emergency Medicine, Oregon Health and Science
University, Portland, Oregon

DAVID M. SPIRO, MD, MPH
Associate Professor, Departments of Emergency Medicine and Pediatrics, Oregon, Health
and Science University, Portland, Oregon

CHARLES R. THOMAS Jr, MD
Professor and Chair, Department of Radiation Medicine, Knight Cancer Institute, Oregon
Health and Science University, Portland, Oregon

AUTHORS

BRUCE D. ADAMS, MD, COL, MC, US ARMY
Chief, Department of Clinical Investigation, William Beaumont Army Medical Center,
El Paso, Texas; Clinical Professor, Department of Emergency Medicine, Medical College
of Georgia, Augusta, Georgia

RUSSELL BAKER, DO
Department of Emergency Medicine, Texas Tech University Heath Sciences Center,
Paul L. Foster School of Medicine, El Paso, Texas

ANDREA BEZJAK, MD, MSc, FRCPC
Associate Professor, Department of Radiation Oncology, University of Toronto, Princess
Margaret Hospital, Toronto, Ontario, Canada

JEFFREY A. BOGART, MD
Professor and Chairman, Department of Radiation Oncology, State University of New York
Upstate Medical University, Syracuse, New York

ROBERT L. CLOUTIER, MD, FAAEM
Assistant Professor of Emergency Medicine and Pediatrics, Department of Emergency Medicine, Doernbecher Children's Hospital, Oregon Health and Science University, Portland, Oregon

RAHUL R. CHOPRA, MD
Department of Radiation Oncology, State University of New York Upstate Medical University, Syracuse, New York

JOY CRANDALL, DO, FACEP, FACMT
Formerly, Senior Resident, Department of Emergency Medicine, Carl R. Darnall Army Medical Center, Fort Hood, Texas; Currently, Brigade Surgeon, 214th Fires Brigade, Reynolds Army Community Hospital Fires Clinic, Fort Sill, Oklahoma

DENISE M. DAMEK, MD
Associate Professor, Neurology and Neurosurgery, University of Colorado Denver School of Medicine, Neuro-Oncology Program, Aurora, Colorado

THOMAS G. DELOUGHERY, MD, FACP
Professor, Division of Hematology and Medical Oncology, Department of Medicine; and Professor, Division of Laboratory Medicine, Department of Pathology; and Professor, Divisions of Hematology and Medical Oncology, Department of Pediatrics, Oregon Health and Science University, Portland, Oregon

PAUL L. DESANDRE, DO
Assistant Professor, Emergency Medicine, Albert Einstein College of Medicine; Attending Physician, Emergency Medicine, Hospice and Palliative Medicine, Beth Israel Medical Center, New York, New York

MELISSA L. GIVENS, MD, MPH
Emergency Medicine Residency Director, Department of Emergency Medicine, Carl R. Darnall Army Medical Center, Fort Hood, Texas; Assistant Professor, Department of Military and Emergency Medicine, Uniformed Services University of the Health Sciences, Bethesda, Maryland

ROBERT F. KACPROWICZ, MD
Program Director, San Antonio Uniformed Services Health Education Consortium Residency in Emergency Medicine, San Antonio, Texas; Assistant Clinical Professor, Department of Emergency Medicine, University of New Mexico School of Medicine, Albuquerque, New Mexico; Department of Emergency Medicine, Wilford Hall USAF Medical Center, Lackland AFB, Texas

JEREMY D. LLOYD, MD
Co-Director of Medical Student and Intern Education, San Antonio Uniformed Services Health Education Consortium Residency in Emergency Medicine, San Antonio; Department of Emergency Medicine, Wilford Hall USAF Medical Center, Lackland AFB, Texas

J. ABRAHAM LOPEZ, MD
Department of Emergency Medicine, Texas Tech University Heath Sciences Center, Paul L. Foster School of Medicine, El Paso, Texas

ANDREW N. NEMECEK, MD
Assistant Professor, Department of Neurological Surgery, Oregon Health and Science University, Portland, Oregon

TAMMIE E. QUEST, MD
Associate Professor, Department of Emergency Medicine, Emory University School of Medicine, Atlanta, Georgia

SUSAN SPENCER, MD
Clinical Assistant Professor, Department of Emergency Medicine, Texas Tech University Heath Sciences Center, Paul L. Foster School of Medicine, El Paso, Texas

HAI SUN, MD, PhD
Resident, Department of Neurological Surgery, Oregon Health and Science University, Portland, Oregon

JONATHAN F. WAN, BASc, MD, FRCPC
Fellow, Department of Radiation Oncology, University of Toronto, Princess Margaret Hospital, Toronto, Ontario; Assistant Professor, Department of Radiation Oncology, McGill University, Montreal General Hospital, Montreal, Quebec, Canada

Contents

Thrombosis is a common complication of cancer, occurring in up to 15% of patients. This article reviews the diagnosis and management of the most common cancer-related thrombotic problems; deep venous thrombosis, pulmonary embolism, and catheter-related thrombosis. Rarer entities, such as cerebral vein thrombosis and Budd-Chiari syndrome, are also reviewed.

Superior vena cava syndrome is a common complication of malignancy. The epidemiology, presentation, and diagnostic evaluation of patients presenting with the syndrome are reviewed. Management options including chemotherapy and radiation therapy and the role of endovascular stents are discussed along with the evidence for each of the therapeutic options.

Neurologic symptoms commonly occur in oncology patients, and in some cases they may be the presenting symptom of malignancy. Cancer-related neurologic syndromes are rarely pathognomonic and must be differentiated from other benign or serious conditions. This article reviews common neuro-oncologic syndromes that may lead to urgent evaluation in the emergency department, including cerebral edema, altered mental status, seizures, acute stroke, leptomeningeal metastases, and paraneoplastic neurologic syndromes.

Malignant epidural spinal cord compression (MESCC) is a common neurologic complication of cancer. MESCC is a medical emergency that needs rapid diagnosis and treatment to prevent undergo emergent evaluation including magnetic resonance imaging of the entire spine. If MESCC is diagnosed, corticosteroids should be administered. Simultaneously, spine surgery and oncology teams should be immediately consulted. If indicated, patients should undergo maximal tumor resection and stabilization, followed by postoperative radiotherapy. Emerging treatment options such as stereotactic radiosurgery and vertebroplasty may be able to provide some symptomatic relief for patients who are not surgical candidates.

A thorough working knowledge of the diagnosis and treatment of life-threatening electrolyte abnormalities in cancer patients, especially hyponatremia, hypoglycemia, and hypercalcemia, is essential to the successful practice of emergency medicine. Although most minor abnormalities have no specific treatment, severe clinical manifestations of several notable electrolytes occur with significant frequency in the setting of malignancy. The treatment of life-threatening electrolyte abnormalities is reviewed here. Promising future treatments directed at the underlying physiology are also introduced.

Acute renal failure (ARF) can be one of the many complications associated with malignancy and, unfortunately, often harbors a worse prognosis for the afflicted patient. Insult to the kidneys can occur for a variety of reasons in the oncologic patient. This article focuses on several of these etiologies, such as tumor lysis syndrome (TLS) and thrombotic microangiopathy (TMA), which are unique threats faced by the oncologic patient.

Neutropenic enterocolitis, also known as typhlitis or ileocecal syndrome, is a rare, but important, complication of neutropenia associated with malignancy. It occurs as a result of chemotherapeutic damage to the intestinal mucosa in the context of an absolute neutropenia and can rapidly progress to intestinal perforation, multisystem organ failure, and sepsis. Presenting signs and symptoms may include fever, abdominal pain, nausea, vomiting, and diarrhea. Rapid identification and timely, aggressive medical and/or surgical intervention are the cornerstones of survival for these patients.

Myeloproliferative disorders and the serum hyperviscosity syndrome can rapidly manifest with emergent presentations. Hyperviscosity occurs from pathologic elevations of either the cellular or acellular (protein) fractions of the circulating blood. Classic hyperviscosity syndrome presents with the triad of bleeding diathesis, visual disturbances, and focal neurologic signs. Emergency medicine providers should be aware of these conditions and be prepared to rapidly initiate supportive and early definitive management, including plasma exchange and apharesis. Early consultation with a hematologist is essential to managing these complex patients.

THE CLINICS ARE NOW AVAILABLE ONLINE!

Access your subscription at:
www.theclinics.com

Preface

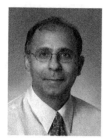 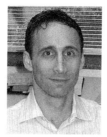 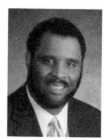

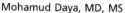

Mohamud Daya, MD, MS   David M. Spiro, MD, MPH   Charles R. Thomas Jr, MD
Guest Editors

Cancer is the second leading cause of death in the United States and affects 1 in 3 people at some point in their lifetime. This issue of the *Hematology/Oncology Clinics of North America* is dedicated to the diagnosis and treatment of cancer-related emergencies. The 11 articles in this issue were previously published as part of a 2-volume series in the *Emergency Medicine Clinics of North America* in 2009. Articles focus on specific presentation syndromes, such as malignant epidural spinal cord compression and superior vena cava (SVC) syndrome. These articles update readers on evidence-based therapies for these entities and highlight the emerging role of stenting as a therapeutic option for SVC syndrome. Also included are articles that address the neurologic, renal, and electrolyte complications encountered in cancer patients. Of particular interest are novel pharmacologic therapies developed for the treatment of tumor lysis syndrome and the syndrome of inappropriate antidiuretic hormone secretion. Various hematologic complications of malignancy, including myeloproliferation/hyperviscosity, venous thrombosis, and acquired bleeding disorders, are also addressed through evidence-based reviews. The issue has dedicated articles that review the toxicities associated with radiation therapy and the challenges associated with diagnosis and treatment of neutropenic enterocolitis. Finally, the important topic of pain management is comprehensively reviewed using the World Health Organization template as a basis. It has been a distinct pleasure to coedit this volume, and we thank all the authors for their outstanding contributions. We also thank the leadership team associated with the *Hematology/Oncology Clinics of North America*, especially Jeannette Forcina, Patrick Manley, and Kerry Holland, for their guidance and

Hematol Oncol Clin N Am 24 (2010) xi–xii
doi:10.1016/j.hoc.2010.03.012
0889-8588/10/$ – see front matter © 2010 Elsevier Inc. All rights reserved.

assistance. Finally, we wish to thank our patients—who continually teach us humility as physicians as we strive toward a better understanding of medicine.

Mohamud Daya, MD, MS
Department of Emergency Medicine
Oregon Health & Science University
3181 SW Sam Jackson Park Road
Mail Code CDW-EM
Portland, OR 97239-3098, USA

David M. Spiro, MD, MPH
Department of Emergency Medicine and Pediatrics
Oregon Health & Science University
3181 SW Sam Jackson Park Road
Mail Code CDW-EM
Portland, OR 97239-3098, USA

Charles R. Thomas Jr, MD
Department of Radiation Medicine
Knight Cancer Institute
Oregon Health & Science University
Mail Code KPV4, 3181 SW Sam Jackson Park Road
Mail Code CDW-EM
Portland, OR 97239-3098, USA

E-mail addresses:
dayam@ohsu.edu (M. Daya)
spirod@ohsu.edu (D.M. Spiro)
thomasch@ohsu.edu (C.R. Thomas)

Erratum

Please note that a clarification is needed in the article entitled, "Inherited Predisposition to Gastrointestinal Stromal Tumor," by Drs Rinki Agarwal and Mark Robson, which published in the February 2009 issue of *Hematology/Oncology Clinics of North America* (23:1). The authors stated mistakenly that the term *Carney-Stratakis syndrome* was coined by Drs Carney and Stratakis to describe patients with an apparent autosomal dominant predisposition to paraganglioma and gastric stromal sarcoma. The authors would like to clarify that the eponym was first proposed by Drs Daum, Vanecek, Sima, and Michel in Gastrointestinal Stromal Tumor: Update. Klinicka Onkologie 2006;19:203–211.

Hematol Oncol Clin N Am 24 (2010) xiii
doi:10.1016/j.hoc.2010.04.001
0889-8588/10/$ – see front matter © 2010 Elsevier Inc. All rights reserved.

Erratum

Venous Thrombotic Emergencies

Thomas G. DeLoughery, MD[a,b,c,*]

KEYWORDS

- Venous thromboembolism • Cancer • Thrombosis
- Anticoagulation • Low–molecular weight heparin • Warfarin

PULMONARY EMBOLISM/DEEP VENOUS THROMBOSIS
Natural History

It is estimated that pulmonary emboli occur in at least 0.5 to 1 per 1000 people in the United States per year, leading to at least 50,000 to 100,000 deaths.[1] More than 90% of pulmonary emboli occur as a complication of thrombosis in the deep venous system of the legs. Therefore, treatment and prevention of deep venous thrombosis (DVT) will reduce the occurrence of pulmonary embolism (PE). Another key point is that more than 90% of the deaths from PE occur within the first hour. Thus, management is aimed at prevention of a repeat embolism and not treatment of the initial embolus. Every aspect of this risk is magnified in patients with cancer, because they are more likely to have thrombosis, more likely to die of their thrombosis, and more likely to have complications of antithrombotic therapy.

Pathophysiology

Cancer patients may develop thrombosis for multiple reasons[2]: in some, the tumor itself expresses procoagulant proteins, such as tissue factor, which directly activate coagulation; in some, large, bulky tumors, such as lymphoma, can cause obstruction of the venous system; and many have high levels of inflammatory cytokines that can directly activate the coagulation system.

Another major etiology of cancer-related thrombosis is therapy. The presence of cancer triples the risk of thrombosis in any surgery. It is estimated that in brain surgery

A version of this article was previously published in the *Emergency Medicine Clinics of North America*, 27:3.

[a] Division of Hematology and Medical Oncology, Department of Medicine, Oregon Health & Science University, L586, 3181 SW Sam Jackson Park Road, Portland, OR 97201-3098, USA
[b] Division of Laboratory Medicine, Department of Pathology, Oregon Health & Science University, 3181 SW Sam Jackson Park Road, Portland, OR 97201-3098, USA
[c] Divisions of Hematology and Medical Oncology, Department of Pediatrics, Oregon Health & Science University, 3181 SW Sam Jackson Park Road, Portland, OR 97201-3098, USA
* Division of Hematology and Medical Oncology, Department of Medicine, Oregon Health & Science University, L586, 3181 SW Sam Jackson Park Road, Portland, OR 97201-3098.
E-mail address: delought@Ohsu.edu

for malignant tumors, as many as 60% of patients will develop thrombosis. This increased risk of thrombosis can be present for up to 6 weeks after surgery.[3]

Chemotherapy can also increase the risk of thrombosis. Early studies showed that receiving adjuvant therapy for breast cancer resulted in a 6.5-fold increase in thrombosis.[4,5] The newer angiogenesis inhibitors, such as thalidomide, sunitinib, and bevacizumab, have marked thrombotic risks. For example, without prophylaxis, 25% of patients receiving thalidomide and chemotherapy developed thrombosis.[6] Finally, all forms of hormonal therapy of breast cancer are associated with a 2- to 3-fold increased risk of thrombosis.[7]

Diagnostic Tests

Patients most often first notice dyspnea and cough after a PE. Chest pain occurs hours to days after the event, with the development of lung infarction. Less than one-third of patients will have hemoptysis, and 10% to 20% will have syncope. Most patients, on examination, will have tachypnea (70%–92%), but less than half have tachycardia. Chest radiographs are normal in only 30% of patients with PE. A nonspecific infiltrate is seen in 50% to 70% of patients with PE and an effusion in 35% of patients with PE. In recent studies, 15% to 30% of patients had partial pressure of oxygen (Po_2) greater than 90 mm Hg, and 20% to 30% had alveolar-arterial gradients less than 20 mm Hg. These results demonstrate that patients with PE need not be hypoxic or have an abnormal a-A gradient.[8,9]

Recently, there has been great interest in clinical prediction rules for DVT and PE. Using these rules, clinicians can better predict which patients are at a higher risk for thrombosis. Validated rules for DVT and PE are summarized in **Tables 1** and **2**. Of note, active cancer is an important component of each of these rules. Use of these prediction rules helps risk-stratify patients and aids in determining the sequence of diagnostic tests.

A major advance in the evaluation of patients with DVT/PE is the wide availability of rapid D-dimer assays.[10] Thrombi have areas that are growing and other areas that are undergoing fibrinolysis. One of the breakdown products of thrombi is called a "D-dimer" whose levels reflect the thrombus burden. All patients with clinically significant thrombosis will have levels of D-dimers above the assay cutoff, thus making it a sensitive screening test for thrombosis. Confusion arises because there are three different types of D-dimer assays available, all with different abilities to help in diagnosing DVT/PE.

Table 1
Wells deep venous thrombosis prediction model

Variable	Points
Active cancer	+1
Paralysis or recent plaster immobilization of lower extremity	+1
Recently bedridden for >3 d or major surgery within 4 wk	+1
Local tenderness CM	+1
Calf swelling >3 cm than asymptomatic side (measured 10 cm below tibial tuberosity)	+1
Pitting edema in symptomatic leg	+1
Dilated superficial veins (nonvaricose) in symptomatic leg only	+1
Alternative diagnoses as or more likely than DVT	−2

Low probability <0, (DVT rate = 3%), moderate probability 1–2 (17%), and high probability >3 (75%).
   Data from Anand SS, Wells PS, Hunt D, et al. Does this patient have deep vein thrombosis? JAMA 1998;279(14):1094–9.

Table 2
Clinical probability score for pulmonary embolism

Wells: Variable	Points
Clinical signs and symptoms of DVT	+3
PE as likely or more likely than alternative diagnosis	+3
Immobilization or surgery in past 4 wk	1.5
Previous PE or DVT	1.5
Heart rate more than 100 beats/min	1.5
Hemoptysis	1
Active cancer	1

Low probability, <2; intermediate probability, 2–6; high probability, >6.

Geneva: Variable	Points
Previous DVT or PE	+1
Recent surgery	+1
Age >65 y	+1
Cancer	+1
Unilateral lower limb pain	+1
Hemoptysis	+1
Heart rate (beats/min)	
75–94	+1
≥95	+1
Pain on lower limb palpation and unilateral edema	+1

Probability: low, 0–4; intermediate, 5–8; high, >9.

	% of Total Patients		% with PE	
Probability of PE	Wells	Geneva	Wells	Geneva
Low	57	36	3.6–7.1	7.7
Medium	36	60	18–25	29.4
High	7	4	50–66	64.3

Data from Gibson NS, Sohne M, Kruip MJ, et al. Further validation and simplification of the Wells clinical decision rule in pulmonary embolism. Thromb Haemost 2008;99(1):229–34; Klok FA, Mos IC, Nijkeuter M, et al. Simplification of the revised Geneva score for assessing clinical probability of pulmonary embolism. Arch Intern Med 2008;168(19):2131–6.

- Latex agglutinin—used for the diagnosis of disseminated intravascular coagulation and usually reported as a titer (for example, "2–4"); lacks sufficient sensitivity to be used as a test in thrombosis.
- Point-of-care D-dimer test—offers binary "yes-no" results[11]; has higher sensitivity, but must be used with decision rules. Most studies show that the combination of a negative point-of-care D-dimer test and a low-probability result on a prediction rule is sufficient to rule out thrombosis without the need for imaging.
- "High-sensitivity" D-dimer test—sensitivity approaches 95%.[10] Combination of a negative D-dimer test and a low-probability result on a prediction rule is sufficient to rule out thrombosis without the need for imaging.

One drawback of the D-dimer test is its lack of specificity, coupled with its high sensitivity. Therefore, patients with positive D-dimer assays require further testing to establish the presence of thrombosis. Patients with recent trauma, recent surgery, pregnancy, or who are older than 70 years have a higher baseline D-dimer level, which greatly limits the use of D-dimers in these patients.[10] Cancer patients also have a higher incidence of increased D-dimer levels; however, there are still a reasonable percentage of patients with negative D-dimers (9%–15%), which makes the test useful for screening patients.[12]

Currently the standard for definite diagnosis of PE is CT angiography (CTA) of the chest.[13–15] Diagnostic approaches that use only CTA have excellent outcomes when compared with those that combine CTA with leg studies or other imaging modalities.[16–18] Sensitivity and specificity are higher for embolism in the segmental and larger blood vessels. Controversy continues over the clinical implications of isolated subsegmental PE because of this being a common finding and the lack of specificity of this finding.[19] A growing concern regarding CTA is the potential overuse of this test and exposure to unnecessary radiation. In many institutions, the positive rate of CTA for embolism is only 5% to 10%. Radiation exposure from a CTA can be equivalent to 100 to 400 chest radiograms or 10 to 30 mammograms, which highlights the need for a structured approach to PE diagnosis.[20]

One issue that has occurred since the widespread use of CTA is the finding of an "unexpected" PE on a CT scan done for another reason, such as cancer screening. In retrospect, many of these patients were having symptoms, such as increased dyspnea.[21] Patients with unexpected PE on CT have increased mortality and need to be treated as aggressively as any patient with PE.[22]

Ventilation perfusion scans are sensitive but not specific for PE.[23] The use of these tests has declined dramatically in the past decade, making it difficult to readily obtain these tests and raising concerns about reliability of interpretation. Only a normal scan rules out embolism, and positive scans have to be interpreted with the patient's pretest probability of thrombosis along with the pattern of the scan. Pulmonary angiography is the gold standard for diagnosis of PE but is rarely performed in the modern era.

Doppler ultrasound is the definitive diagnostic test in patients with symptoms of DVT.[24] Sensitivity and specificity are greater than 95% for lower-extremity thrombosis. Use of venography or CT may be appropriate in patients with a high suspicion of thrombosis but with a negative ultrasound.

Diagnostic pathways
Deep venous thrombosis Pretest probability should be determined using the Wells rule. If a high probability of DVT is not present, then the emergency physician should obtain a high-sensitivity D-dimer test. If the D-dimer level is normal, an alternative diagnosis needs to be considered, and no further testing is needed for thrombosis. If the patient has a high probability score or positive D-dimer test, then a Doppler examination is performed. If the Doppler is positive for thrombosis, anticoagulation therapy should be started immediately in the emergency department (ED) (**Fig. 1**).

Pulmonary embolism Pretest probability should be determined using the Wells or Geneva rules. If a high probability of DVT is not present, then the emergency physician should obtain a high-sensitivity D-dimer. If the D-dimer is normal, an alternative diagnosis needs to be considered, and no further testing is needed for thrombosis. If the patient has a high-probability score or positive D-dimer, then a CTA is performed and, if positive, anticoagulation therapy is started in the ED.

Immediate Therapy of Thrombosis

Thrombolytic therapy
Given the natural history of PE, the role of thrombolytic therapy is uncertain.[25–28] The fact that thrombolytic therapy lyses clots faster than heparin seems to be of no

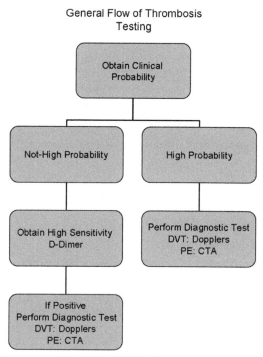

Fig. 1. Algorithm for approach to DVT and PE in the emergency department.

long-term clinical significance in most patients. Even in patients with PE associated with right ventricular dysfunction, use of thrombolytic therapy failed to show an improvement in death rates.[29] Many patients with PE are poor candidates for thrombolytic therapy due to recent surgery or other reasons. Also of concern is the 1% to 2% risk of intracranial hemorrhage that accompanies thrombolytic therapy.[30] The vast majority of patients with PE who survive long enough to be diagnosed with their embolism will probably survive the acute event. Their increased delayed mortality with PE is mainly due to underlying diseases, such as cancer. Therefore, only a small number of patients would benefit from thrombolytic therapy. However, fibrinolytic therapy remains an option for the patient in extremis because of a PE who is not a candidate for embolectomy (**Box 1**).

If thrombolytic therapy is required, the dosing for the medications is the same as that for cardiac indications. Plasma fibrinogen and activated partial thromboplastin time (aPTT) should be measured every 4 hours after treatment. If the aPTT is below two times normal and the fibrinogen is more than 100 mg/dL, heparin should be started.[26,31]

Intravenous thrombolytic therapy for DVT has little effect on long-term outcomes, such as post-phlebitic syndrome.[32] It therefore has little role in the management of these patients. One area where thrombolytic therapy is increasingly useful is when using catheter-guided lytic therapy to recanalize the vein in massive DVT, involving the common femoral or iliac system.[33] Often, these patients with underlying venous compression can also have venous stenting or vasoplasty to fix the lesions during catheterization.

Surgical embolectomy may be useful in the small subset of patients who are in unresponsive shock. Some series claim up to 70% survival.[34] A patient may be a candidate

---

Box 1
Summary of therapy options for venous thromboembolic disease

Immediate therapy

Thrombolytic therapy

    Pulmonary embolism: consider in patients with refractory hypotension

    Deep venous thrombosis: consider catheter-directed therapy for iliofemoral thrombosis

    Embolectomy: consider in PE patients with cardiac arrest or refractory hypotension

Inferior vena cava filters: consider if patients have a contraindication to anticoagulation therapy

Heparin

    Heparin: bolus 5000 to 10,000 units followed by 1000 to 2000 units/h to achieve heparin levels of 0.35 to 0.7 anti-Xa units

    Low–molecular weight heparin:

        Dalteparin: 100 units/kg every 12 h

        Enoxaparin: 1 mg/kg every 12 h or 1.5 mg/kg in low-risk patients

        Tinzaparin: 175 units every 24 h

        Fondaparinux (pentasaccharide): 7.5 mg every 24 h (5.0 mg in patients weighing less than 50 kg and 10 mg in patients weighing more than 100 kg)

---

for embolectomy if persistent signs of shock remain with a suspected or confirmed massive PE after an hour of medical management in the ED setting. Specific examples of persistent shock in adult patients would include a systolic blood pressure of less than 90 mm Hg, urine output of less than 20 mL/h, or Po_2 of less than 60 mm Hg. This approach requires the presence of a qualified cardiothoracic surgeon.

The role of inferior vena cava filters in the treatment of thromboembolic disease is unclear because of a lack of good trials.[32,35] A strong indication for filter placement would be PE with DVT in a patient in whom anticoagulant therapy is transiently contraindicated. However, a filter is never a replacement for long-term anticoagulation therapy, so even in these patients, anticoagulation therapy needs to be started as soon as feasible. This is especially true in cancer patients; 17% to 66% of those who receive filters instead of anticoagulation therapy will have thrombotic complications.[36–38]

Elastic compression stockings are extremely useful in the prevention of post-phlebitic syndrome. All patients with DVT should be prescribed knee-high stockings with the compression "dose" being 30 to 40 mm Hg at the ankles.[39] Patients should be advised to wear stockings most of the day and everyday for best effect.

There is now abundant evidence that using low–molecular weight heparin (LMWH) for therapy in DVT and PE treatment is just as effective as unfractionated heparin for any type of venous thrombosis, ranging from submassive PE to superficial thrombophlebitis.[32,40–45] There are also data supporting the use of pentasaccharide fondaparinux; however, its long half-life and renal clearance may be concerns in older patients or those with renal problems.[46]

For most patients receiving LMWH therapy, laboratory monitoring is not required. Monitoring should be considered for patients who are very obese (greater than 2 times their ideal body weight), who have severe liver or heart failure, who are pregnant, or who require long-term therapy. Very obese patients still require actual body weight–based dosing without "capping" the dose at an arbitrary level but require a level the second day of therapy.[47] LMWH is cleared by a renal mechanism and will accumulate in patients with renal failure. Therefore, in patients with renal failure, initial dosing should be reduced by 50% and levels monitored. However, the use of LMWH is not associated with an additional risk of bleeding when compared with standard heparin.[48] All patients should receive at least 5 days of heparin therapy. Recommended initial LMWH doses are summarized in **Box 2**.

If used (see later discussion), warfarin is started the evening of initial diagnosis with a loading dose of 2.5 to 10 mg orally; 5 mg is recommended in most patients.[49] Healthy patients younger than 60 years may need a 10-mg loading dose, whereas those older than 85 years, frail and elderly, should start with 2.5 mg.[50] Warfarin is titrated to an international normalized ratio (INR) of 2-3. Use of warfarin affects all the vitamin K–dependent proteins. The first coagulation factor to be reduced by warfarin therapy is factor VII, resulting in prolongation of the INR. However, the full antithrombotic effect of warfarin does not occur until factors X and II levels have decreased. This decrease will take an additional 24 to 48 hours after factor VII levels are reduced. This is the rationale why patients should overlap heparin and warfarin therapy for several days. In patients with acute thrombosis, warfarin should never be started as the sole therapy. Outcomes are superior with the use of heparin before warfarin, and use of warfarin without heparin also puts the patient at risk for warfarin-associated skin necrosis due to interference with protein C and S synthesis.[51]

Duration and Choice of Therapy

Past studies have shown that cancer patients treated with warfarin have 2- to 3-fold higher risk for bleeding and rethrombosis compared with patients who have thrombosis but no cancer.[52] Four studies have shown that cancer patients treated with LMWH have significantly lower rates of recurrent thrombosis but not an increased risk of bleeding and should be considered for treatment for at least 3 months with LMWH.[4,32] This is especially true for patients with pancreatic, brain, or lung cancer.[53] Presence of cancer is a major risk for recurrent thrombosis, and patients should be treated until they are cancer-free, or lifelong in the presence of metastatic disease. Patients on warfarin who have recurrent thrombosis need to be changed to indefinite LMWH therapy.

SPECIAL THROMBOSIS ISSUES IN CANCER PATIENTS
Thrombosis in Patients with Primary Brain Tumors or Metastases

The presence of brain tumors markedly increases the risk of thrombosis. There is often concern about the risk of hemorrhage into the brain if anticoagulation therapy is used. However, this risk is very low for most patients. One study in glioma patients showed identical rates of intracranial hemorrhage in patients on and off anticoagulation

Box 2
Hypercoagulable states associated with Budd-Chiari syndrome
Antiphospholipid antibodies
Behçet syndrome
Myeloproliferative syndrome
Paroxysmal nocturnal hemoglobinuria

therapy.[54] However, patients with brain metastases from choriocarcinoma, melanoma, renal, and thyroid cancer should not be treated with an anticoagulant because of high rates of spontaneous bleeding seen with these tumors.[55] For patients with other tumors, a brain CT should be obtained first to rule out the presence of bleeding before initiating therapy.

Anticoagulation and Thrombocytopenia

Concern regarding the use of anticoagulation therapy in the presence of thrombocytopenia is a valid apprehension; however, scant data exist to guide therapy. A reasonable approach is no anticoagulation at therapeutic dosages when the platelet count is less than 50,000/µL. This is based on indirect data from hemophiliacs, which showed that a platelet count less than 50,000/µL was associated with a marked increase in bleeding.[56] Any form of anticoagulation should be stopped when the count decreases to less than 20,000/µL.

Upper-Extremity Thrombosis

Central venous catheters (CVCs) are essential to many aspects of cancer therapy. The clinically apparent thrombosis incidence for catheters is estimated to be 5% to 30% and can be as high as 40% with peripherally inserted central catheters (PICCs).[29,57] The signs of catheter thrombosis are nonspecific, and the incidence of thrombosis is thought to be underestimated. CVCs are often coated with sheaths of fibrin soon after introduction. Catheter thrombosis can also be a sign of heparin-induced thrombocytopenia (HIT), because heparin is often used to ensure patency. Unlike lower-extremity thrombosis, the incidence of PE with upper-extremity thrombosis is much lower—only 8% versus 31% in one study.[58]

Therapy starts with removing the catheter, because this will remove the nidus of thrombus. If the patient is not at risk for bleeding, one should consider anticoagulation therapy for 4 to 6 weeks. One can try to "salvage" the catheter by anticoagulating the patients while maintaining the catheter in place, but this approach was associated with a 4% incidence of serious bleeding in a pilot study. Given the low risk of long-term sequelae, there is little indication for thrombolytic therapy.

Prevention of catheter thrombosis is controversial.[59] Most studies have not shown a benefit to prophylaxis against thrombosis with LMWH or warfarin.

Cerebral Vein Thrombosis

Cerebral vein thrombosis occurs commonly in the cerebral sinuses, but in some cases it occurs in the deep cerebral veins.[60] One of the risk factors for thrombosis is the presence of venous hypercoagulable states, including malignancies. Patients with acquired hypercoagulable states, such as paroxysmal nocturnal hemoglobinuria (PNH) or myeloproliferative syndromes, seem to be at increased risk. Another group of patients at risk are those suffering from severe dehydration with sludging of the cerebral blood flow. Finally, patients may have thrombosis due to local irritation of the venous sinuses. The classic presentation of infection-related thrombosis is a cerebral vein thrombosis due to irritation of the transverse sinus by mastoiditis, which is also called "otic hydrocephalus."

Patients with cerebral vein thrombosis can present with one of two major patterns.[61] The first is with focal neurologic defects due to venous thrombosis, resulting in localized infarction. Infarctions are often hemorrhagic due to continued arterial blood flow, which pumps blood into the infarcted area. Patients with cerebral vein thrombosis will usually present with signs of increased intracranial pressure due to obstruction of venous flow and cerebrospinal fluid reabsorption. Patients will often have severe headaches, nausea, and vomiting and may then progress to coma due to infarction of deep brain structures. Patients may also have reduced vision and blindness due to pressure on the optic nerve. Frequently, patients have a prolonged course lasting for days, with gradual worsening of symptoms.

Especially early in the course of cerebral vein thrombosis, patients may present with nonspecific signs and symptoms. Often patients may be misdiagnosed as having pseudotumor cerebri. This misdiagnosis may occur if only CT scanning is done and found to be normal and the lumbar puncture demonstrates high opening pressures. Diagnosis of cerebral vein thrombosis is best made by MRI and MR angiography, which may best show the venous obstruction.

Cerebral vein thrombosis requires anticoagulation. Despite the frequent presence of hemorrhagic transformation, immediate heparin therapy is associated with an improvement in outcome. In the Einhäupl trial, when patients received a small 3000-unit bolus of heparin, a dramatic improvement in outcome was seen compared with controls.[62] Currently, immediate therapy with either standard heparin or LMWH followed by warfarin is the recommended antithrombotic therapy.[63,64] Patients with severe neurologic deficits may benefit from angiography and direct thrombolytic therapy of the venous obstruction. Patients with mastoiditis or other local infections should be given anticoagulation therapy for 6 months. Patients with idiopathic thrombosis or cancer-related causes should be given anticoagulation therapy indefinitely.[64]

Adrenal Infarction

The adrenal gland contains a plexus of small veins and venules that receive the secreted hormones of the adrenal gland. This venous structure seems to be prone to thrombosis in several hypercoagulable states. Patients with purpura fulminans may present with adrenal crisis due to thrombosis and the resultant hemorrhagic destruction of the adrenal gland. Patients with HIT may rarely infarct the gland and have subsequent hemorrhage.[65] Finally, patients with the antiphospholipid antibody syndrome (APLS) can have adrenal infarctions. The presentation in APLS patients is often one of adrenal insufficiency that may be overlooked initially due to nonspecific symptoms.[66]

Budd-Chiari Syndrome

Patients with Budd-Chiari syndrome or hepatic vein thrombosis present with the onset of a painful swollen liver and ascites that may progress to liver failure.[67,68] Several hypercoagulable states are associated with Budd-Chiari syndrome (see **Box 2**), which include the myeloproliferative syndromes—APLS, PNH, and Behçet syndrome. Budd-Chiari syndrome may be the presenting sign of a myeloproliferative syndrome and can occur with normal blood counts.[69]

Therapy is partially dictated by the severity of the liver disease. Because these patients have a hypercoagulable state and are at risk for further life-threatening thrombosis, anticoagulation should be initiated at the time of diagnosis of the thrombosis. Patients who present acutely may be treated with catheter-guided thrombolytic therapy. Patients who present with chronic obstruction may benefit from either surgical or catheter-placed shunts. Patients with hepatic vein thrombosis due to myeloproliferative syndromes do poorly with surgery; therefore, catheter-based shunt approaches should be initially attempted. Despite the presence of hypercoagulable states, shunt thrombosis is uncommon if the patient is given anticoagulation therapy. Patients who undergo liver transplantation and have an identifiable hypercoagulable state should be aggressively anticoagulated to prevent thrombosis of the liver graft.[70]

Portal Vein Thrombosis

With the increase in noninvasive imaging of the abdomen, the incidence of portal vein thrombosis is also increasing. The risk factors for idiopathic portal vein thrombosis are similar to those for Budd-Chiari syndrome.[71] Increasingly, portal vein thrombosis is being recognized as a complication of upper abdominal surgery and laparoscopic colectomy.[72,73] Patient presentation can range from mild abdominal pain to infraction of the bowel and associated symptoms of an acute abdomen. Data suggest that in provoked portal vein thrombosis, aggressive anticoagulation therapy will aid in the recanalization of the portal vein, and so 3 to 6 months of therapy is reasonable.[74] Patients with idiopathic portal vein thrombosis should be given anticoagulation therapy indefinitely.

Renal Vein Thrombosis

Renal vein thrombosis is most commonly associated with nephrotic syndrome. It is also associated with malignancy but is seen less often with the inherited hypercoagulable states. Patients can present with a clinical spectrum ranging from sudden onset of severe flank pain to a subtle deterioration of renal function.[75] Patients with preexisting renal disease may simply present with worsening renal function. Total venous occlusion will result In hemorrhagic infarction of the entire kidney. Acute thrombosis resulting in renal impairment can be treated with catheter-guided thrombolytic therapy. Patients with more chronic presentations require long-term anticoagulation therapy.

Visceral Vein Thrombosis

DVT and cerebral vein thrombosis are the two most common presentations of hypercoagulable states. Mesenteric veins are the third most common presenting site of thrombosis.[76] Patients usually present with abdominal pain out of proportion to physical findings. Diagnosis can be established at the time of surgery or with CT scanning showing thrombus in the mesenteric vein. Patients may experience extensive bowel infarction with mesenteric vein thrombosis.[77] Once identified, patients with mesenteric vein thrombosis should be treated indefinitely with anticoagulation, even in the absence of an identifiable hypercoagulable state, because this condition has a strong association with recurrent thrombosis.

SUMMARY

Patients with cancer pose many challenges for the ED physician, ranging from the increased incidence of thrombosis to presentation at unusual sites. Suspicion needs to be high in cancer patients for the presence of thrombosis, especially in atypical sites. The mainstay of therapy is LMWH, and antithrombotic therapy needs to be continued as long as a tumor is present.

REFERENCES

1. Laack TA, Goyal DG. Pulmonary embolism: an unsuspected killer. Emerg Med Clin North Am 2004;22(4):961–83.
2. Lee AY. Cancer and thromboembolic disease: pathogenic mechanisms. Cancer Treat Rev 2002;28(3):137–40.
3. Geerts WH, Bergqvist D, Pineo GF, et al. Prevention of venous thromboembolism: American College of Chest Physicians Evidence-Based Clinical Practice Guidelines. (8th edition). Chest 2008;133(6 Suppl):381S–453S.

4. Lyman GH, Khorana AA, Falanga A, et al. American Society of Clinical Oncology guideline: recommendations for venous thromboembolism prophylaxis and treatment in patients with cancer. J Clin Oncol 2007;25(34):5490–505.
5. Rella C, Coviello M, Giotta F, et al. A prothrombotic state in breast cancer patients treated with adjuvant chemotherapy. Breast Cancer Res Treat 1996;40(2):151–9.
6. Hussein MA. Thromboembolism risk reduction in multiple myeloma patients treated with immunomodulatory drug combinations. Thromb Haemost 2006; 95(6):924–30.
7. Lycette JL, Luoh SW, Beer TM, et al. Acute bilateral pulmonary emboli occurring while on adjuvant aromatase inhibitor therapy with anastrozole: case report and review of the literature. Breast Cancer Res Treat 2006;99(3):249–55.
8. Stein PD, Beemath A, Matta F, et al. Clinical characteristics of patients with acute pulmonary embolism: data from PIOPED II. Am J Med 2007;120(10):871–9.
9. Stein PD, Fowler SE, Goodman LR, et al. Multidetector computed tomography for acute pulmonary embolism. N Engl J Med 2006;354(22):2317–27.
10. Righini M, Perrier A, De MP, et al. D-dimer for venous thromboembolism diagnosis: 20 years later. J Thromb Haemost 2008;6(7):1059–71.
11. Chunilal SD, Brill-Edwards PA, Stevens PB, et al. The sensitivity and specificity of a red blood cell agglutination D-dimer assay for venous thromboembolism when performed on venous blood. Arch Intern Med 2002;162(2):217–20.
12. King V, Vaze AA, Moskowitz CS, et al. D-dimer assay to exclude pulmonary embolism in high-risk oncologic population: correlation with CT pulmonary angiography in an urgent care setting. Radiology 2008;247(3):854–61.
13. Schoepf UJ, Goldhaber SZ, Costello P. Spiral computed tomography for acute pulmonary embolism. Circulation 2004;109(18):2160–7.
14. Schoepf UJ, Costello P. CT angiography for diagnosis of pulmonary embolism: state of the art. Radiology 2004;230(2):329–37.
15. Donato AA, Scheirer JJ, Atwell MS, et al. Clinical outcomes in patients with suspected acute pulmonary embolism and negative helical computed tomographic results in whom anticoagulation was withheld. Arch Intern Med 2003;163(17):2033–8.
16. British Thoracic Society guidelines for the management of suspected acute pulmonary embolism. Thorax 2003;58(6):470–83.
17. Prologo JD, Gilkeson RC, Diaz M, et al. The effect of single-detector CT versus MDCT on clinical outcomes in patients with suspected acute pulmonary embolism and negative results on CT pulmonary angiography. AJR Am J Roentgenol 2005;184(4):1231–5.
18. Righini M, Le GG, Aujesky D, et al. Diagnosis of pulmonary embolism by multidetector CT alone or combined with venous ultrasonography of the leg: a randomised non-inferiority trial. Lancet 2008;371(9621):1343–52.
19. Konstantinides SV. Acute pulmonary embolism revisited: thromboembolic venous disease. Heart 2008;94(6):795–802.
20. Parker MS, Hui FK, Camacho MA, et al. Female breast radiation exposure during CT pulmonary angiography. AJR Am J Roentgenol 2005;185(5):1228–33.
21. O'Connell CL, Boswell WD, Duddalwar V, et al. Unsuspected pulmonary emboli in cancer patients: clinical correlates and relevance. J Clin Oncol 2006;24(30): 4928–32.
22. O'Connell CL, Ghalichi M, Boyle S, et al. Unsuspected pulmonary emboli identified on routine cancer staging MDCT scans: impact on cancer survival. ASH Annual Meeting Abstracts 2008;112(11):3818.
23. Anderson DR, Kahn SR, Rodger MA, et al. Computed tomographic pulmonary angiography vs ventilation-perfusion lung scanning in patients with suspected

pulmonary embolism: a randomized controlled trial. JAMA 2007;298(23): 2743–53.

24. Segal JB, Eng J, Tamariz LJ, et al. Review of the evidence on diagnosis of deep venous thrombosis and pulmonary embolism. Ann Fam Med 2007;5(1):63–73.

25. Arcasoy SM, Kreit JW. Thrombolytic therapy of pulmonary embolism—a comprehensive review of current evidence. Chest 1999;115(6):1695–707.

26. Riedel M. Acute pulmonary embolism 2: treatment. Heart 2001;85:351–60.

27. Wan S, Quinlan DJ, Agnelli G, et al. Thrombolysis compared with heparin for the initial treatment of pulmonary embolism: a meta-analysis of the randomized controlled trials. Circulation 2004;110(6):744–9.

28. Worster A, Smith C, Silver S, et al. Evidence-based emergency medicine/critically appraised topic. Thrombolytic therapy for submassive pulmonary embolism? Ann Emerg Med 2007;50(1):78–84.

29. Konstantinides S, Geibel A, Heusel G, et al. Heparin plus alteplase compared with heparin alone in patients with submassive pulmonary embolism. N Engl J Med 2002;347(15):1143–50.

30. Kanter DS, Mikkola KM, Patel SR, et al. Thrombolytic therapy for pulmonary embolism—frequency of intracranial hemorrhage and associated risk factors. Chest 1997;111:1241–5.

31. Tapson VF. Acute pulmonary embolism. N Engl J Med 2008;358(10):1037–52.

32. Kearon C, Kahn SR, Agnelli G, et al. Antithrombotic therapy for venous thromboembolic disease: American College of Chest Physicians Evidence-Based Clinical Practice Guidelines. (8th edition). Chest 2008;133(6 Suppl):454S–545S.

33. Comerota AJ, Gravett MH. Iliofemoral venous thrombosis. J Vasc Surg 2007; 46(5):1065–76.

34. Gulba DC, Schmid C, Borst H-G, et al. Medical compared with surgical treatment for massive pulmonary embolism. Lancet 1994;343:576–7.

35. Chung J, Owen RJ. Using inferior vena cava filters to prevent pulmonary embolism. Can Fam Physician 2008;54(1):49–55.

36. Ihnat DM, Mills JL, Hughes JD, et al. Treatment of patients with venous thromboembolism and malignant disease: should vena cava filter placement be routine? J Vasc Surg 1998;28(5):800–7.

37. Levin JM, Schiff D, Loeffler JS, et al. Complications of therapy for venous thromboembolic disease in patients with brain tumors. Neurology 1993;43(6): 1111–4.

38. Schiff D, DeAngelis LM. Therapy of venous thromboembolism in patients with brain metastases. Cancer 1994;73:493–8.

39. Prandoni P, Lensing AW, Prins MH, et al. Below-knee elastic compression stockings to prevent the post-thrombotic syndrome: a randomized, controlled trial. Ann Intern Med 2004;141(4):249–56.

40. Koopman MMW, Prandoni P, Piovella F, et al. Treatment of venous thrombosis with intravenous unfractionated heparin administered in the hospital as compared with subcutaneous low-molecular-weight heparin administered at home. N Engl J Med 1996;334:682–7.

41. Raskob GE. Heparin and low molecular weight heparin for treatment of acute pulmonary embolism [see comments]. Curr Opin Pulm Med 1999;5(4):216–21.

42. Pineo GF, Hull RD. Heparin and low-molecular-weight heparin in the treatment of venous thromboembolism. Baillieres Clin Haematol 1998;11(3):621–37.

43. Buller HR, Agnelli G, Hull RD, et al. Antithrombotic therapy for venous thromboembolic disease: the Seventh ACCP Conference on Antithrombotic and Thrombolytic Therapy. Chest 2004;126(3 Suppl):401S–28S.

44. Schutgens RE, Esseboom EU, Snijder RJ, et al. Low molecular weight heparin (dalteparin) is equally effective as unfractionated heparin in reducing coagulation activity and perfusion abnormalities during the early treatment of pulmonary embolism. J Lab Clin Med 2004;144(2):100–7.

45. Quinlan DJ, McQuillan A, Eikelboom JW. Low-molecular-weight heparin compared with intravenous unfractionated heparin for treatment of pulmonary embolism: a meta-analysis of randomized, controlled trials. Ann Intern Med 2004;140(3):175–83.

46. Buller HR, Davidson BL, Decousus H, et al. Subcutaneous fondaparinux versus intravenous unfractionated heparin in the initial treatment of pulmonary embolism. N Engl J Med 2003;349(18):1695–702.

47. Yee JYV, Duffull SB. The effect of body weight on dalteparin pharmacokinetics— a preliminary study. Eur J Clin Pharmacol 2000;56(4):293–7.

48. Lim W, Cook DJ, Crowther MA. Safety and efficacy of low molecular weight heparins for hemodialysis in patients with end-stage renal failure: a meta-analysis of randomized trials. J Am Soc Nephrol 2004;15(12):3192–206.

49. Crowther MA, Ginsberg JB, Kearon C, et al. A randomized trial comparing 5-mg and 10-mg warfarin loading doses. Arch Intern Med 1999;159(1):46–8.

50. Ageno W, Turpie AG, Steidl L, et al. Comparison of a daily fixed 2.5-mg warfarin dose with a 5-mg, international normalized ratio adjusted, warfarin dose initially following heart valve replacement. Am J Cardiol 2001;88(1):40–4.

51. Brandjes DPM, Heijboer H, Büller HR, et al. Acenocoumarol and heparin compared with acenocoumarol alone in the initial treatment of proximal-vein thrombosis. N Engl J Med 1992;327:1485–9.

52. Prandoni P, Lensing AW, Piccioli A, et al. Recurrent venous thromboembolism and bleeding complications during anticoagulant treatment in patients with cancer and venous thrombosis. Blood 2002;100(10):3484–8.

53. Stein PD, Beemath A, Meyers FA, et al. Incidence of venous thromboembolism in patients hospitalized with cancer. Am J Med 2006;119(1):60–8.

54. Ruff RL, Posner JB. Incidence and treatment of peripheral venous thrombosis in patients with glioma. Ann Neurol 1983;13(3):334–6.

55. Gerber DE, Grossman SA, Streiff MB. Management of venous thromboembolism in patients with primary and metastatic brain tumors. J Clin Oncol 2006;24(8):1310–8.

56. Ragni MV, Bontempo FA, Myers DJ, et al. Hemorrhagic sequelae of immune thrombocytopenic purpura in human immunodeficiency virus-infected hemophiliacs. Blood 1990;75(6):1267–72.

57. Cheong K, Perry D, Karapetis C, et al. High rate of complications associated with peripherally inserted central venous catheters in patients with solid tumours. Intern Med J 2004;34(5):234–8.

58. Lechner D, Wiener C, Weltermann A, et al. Comparison between idiopathic deep vein thrombosis of the upper and lower extremity regarding risk factors and recurrence. J Thromb Haemost 2008;6(8):1269–74.

59. Akl EA, Kamath G, Yosuico V, et al. Thromboprophylaxis for patients with cancer and central venous catheters: a systematic review and a meta-analysis. Cancer 2008;112(11):2483–92.

60. Stam J. Cerebral venous and sinus thrombosis: incidence and causes. Adv Neurol 2003;92:225–32.

61. Dentali F, Ageno W. Natural history of cerebral vein thrombosis. Curr Opin Pulm Med 2007;13(5):372–6.

62. Einhäupl KM, Villringer A, Meister W, et al. Heparin treatment in sinus venous thrombosis. Lancet 1991;338:597–600.

63. Stam J, Lensing AW, Vermeulen M, et al. Heparin treatment for cerebral venous and sinus thrombosis. Lancet 1991;338:1154.

64. Albers GW, Amarenco P, Easton JD, et al. Antithrombotic and thrombolytic therapy for ischemic stroke: American College of Chest Physicians Evidence-Based Clinical Practice Guidelines. (8th edition). Chest 2008;133(6 Suppl): 630S–69S.

65. Kurtz LE, Yang S. Bilateral adrenal hemorrhage associated with heparin induced thrombocytopenia. Am J Hematol 2007;82(6):493–4.

66. Inam S, Sidki K, al-Marshedy AR, et al. Addison's disease, hypertension, renal and hepatic microthrombosis in 'primary' antiphospholipid syndrome. Postgrad Med J 1991;67:385–8.

67. Menon KV, Shah V, Kamath PS. The Budd-Chiari syndrome. N Engl J Med 2004; 350(6):578–85.

68. Plessier A, Valla DC. Budd-Chiari syndrome. Semin Liver Dis 2008;28(3):259–69.

69. Janssen HL, Leebeek FW. JAK2 mutation: the best diagnostic tool for myeloproliferative disease in splanchnic vein thrombosis? Hepatology 2006;44(6):1391–3.

70. Halff G, Todo S, Tzakis AG, et al. Liver transplantation for the Budd-Chiari syndrome. Ann Surg 1990;211:43–9.

71. Bayraktar Y, Harmanci O. Etiology and consequences of thrombosis in abdominal vessels. World J Gastroenterol 2006;12(8):1165–74.

72. Preventza OA, Habib FA, Young SC, et al. Portal vein thrombosis: an unusual complication of laparoscopic cholecystectomy. JSLS 2005;9(1):87–90.

73. Poultsides GA, Lewis WC, Feld R, et al. Portal vein thrombosis after laparoscopic colectomy: thrombolytic therapy via the superior mesenteric vein. Am Surg 2005; 71(10):856–60.

74. Spaander VM, Van Buuren HR, Janssen HL. Review article: the management of non-cirrhotic non-malignant portal vein thrombosis and concurrent portal hypertension in adults. Aliment Pharmacol Ther 2007;26(Suppl 2):203–9.

75. Asghar M, Ahmed K, Shah SS, et al. Renal vein thrombosis. Eur J Vasc Endovasc Surg 2007;34(2):217–23.

76. Kumar S, Sarr MG, Kamath PS. Mesenteric venous thrombosis. N Engl J Med 2001;345(23):1683–8.

77. Hassan HA, Raufman JP. Mesenteric venous thrombosis. South Med J 1999; 92(6):558–62.

Superior Vena Cava Syndrome

Jonathan F. Wan, BASc, MD, FRCPC[a,b,*],
Andrea Bezjak, MD, MSc, FRCPC[a]

KEYWORDS

- Superior vena cava syndrome • Cancer
- Superior vena cava obstruction • Radiation therapy
- Endovascular stenting • Chemotherapy

Superior vena cava syndrome (SVCS) is a common complication of malignancy, especially of lung cancer and lymphoma. The frequency of SVCS varies depending on the specific malignancy. Approximately 2% to 4% of all patients with lung cancer develop SVCS at some time during their disease course.[1–6] The incidence is higher in small cell lung cancer (SCLC), given its predilection for mediastinal involvement and rapid growth; the incidence approaches 10%.[5,7,8] SVCS develops in approximately 2% to 4% of non-Hodgkin's lymphoma (NHL)[1,4] but is relatively rare in Hodgkin's lymphoma despite the presence of mediastinal lymphadenopathy.[9] For primary mediastinal large B-cell lymphomas with sclerosis, the incidence has been reported as high as 57% in one series of 30 patients.[10] Together, lung cancer and lymphoma are responsible for over 90% of malignant causes of SVCS.[3,11] In the modern era, 60% to 90% of cases of SVCS are caused by malignant tumors, with the remaining cases accounted for largely by fibrosing mediastinitis and thrombosis of indwelling central venous devices and/or pacemaker leads.[3,12–14] The focus of this article is on the management of malignant causes of SVCS.

ANATOMY AND PHYSIOLOGY

The superior vena cava (SVC) is the major vessel collecting venous return to the heart from the head, arms, and upper torso. Compression of the SVC in malignancy

A version of this article was previously published in the *Emergency Medicine Clinics of North America*, 27:2.

Statement regarding funding/support: Dr Wan received support from the Radiation Oncology Fellowship Program at the Princess Margaret Hospital, University of Toronto.

[a] Department of Radiation Oncology, University of Toronto, Princess Margaret Hospital, 610 University Avenue, Toronto, Ontario, Canada M5G 2M9

[b] Department of Radiation Oncology, McGill University, Montreal General Hospital, 1650 Cedar Avenue, Montreal, Quebec, Canada H3G 1A4

* Corresponding author. Department of Radiation Oncology, University of Toronto, Princess Margaret Hospital, 610 University Avenue, Toronto, Ontario, Canada M5G 2M9.

E-mail address: jonathan.wan@muhc.mcgill.ca

Hematol Oncol Clin N Am 24 (2010) 501–513
doi:10.1016/j.hoc.2010.03.003
0889-8588/10/$ – see front matter © 2010 Elsevier Inc. All rights reserved.

is usually due to extrinsic masses in the middle or anterior mediastinum, right paratracheal or precarinal lymph node stations, and tumors extending from the right upper lobe bronchus. As the tumors increase in size and produce compression of the SVC, there is increased resistance to venous blood flow, which is then diverted through collateral networks that may develop. Collateral vessels that are commonly found include azygos, intercostal, mediastinal, paravertebral, hemiazygos, thoracoepigastric, internal mammary, thoracoacromioclavicular, and anterior chest wall veins.[15] The severity of SVCS is worse if the level of obstruction is below the azygos vein, underscoring the importance of this vessel in providing an alternate route for blood flow.[16] The severity of the obstruction is also dependent on the rapidity of onset of the obstruction. Collateral vessels often take several weeks to dilate sufficiently to accommodate the diverted blood flow of the SVC. The presence of collateral vessels with compression of SVC on computed tomography (CT) is a reliable indicator of the presence of SVCS with a sensitivity of 96% and specificity of 92%.[17]

PRESENTATION

Patients often complain of a variety of symptoms. The most common of these are facial or neck swelling (82%), arm swelling (68%), dyspnea (66%), cough (50%), and dilated chest veins (38%).[11,13] Patients may also report chest pain, dysphagia, hoarseness, headache, confusion, dizziness, and syncope. Orthopnea is commonly noted, since a supine position will increase the amount of blood flow to the upper torso. Attention should be given to the duration of symptoms, previous diagnosis of malignancy, or previous intravascular procedures for clues to the etiology of the syndrome. In most cases, symptoms develop over the course of several weeks allowing for collateral circulations to develop.

Worrisome signs include stridor, as this is usually indicative of laryngeal edema, as well as confusion and obtundation, since these may indicate cerebral edema. Although SVCS is now known not to be a major threat to life in most clinical scenarios, evidence of respiratory and neurologic compromise can be associated with serious or fatal outcomes. In addition, patients may have other cancer-related symptoms, such as extrinsic compression of major airway by tumor (which may be an alternate explanation for the stridor), hemoptysis, or thrombosis associated with malignant SVCS, which may need to be addressed urgently and may be more life threatening. Patients may also have B symptoms (eg, drenching night sweats, weight loss, or fevers usually associated with lymphomas) or other constitutional symptoms.

In the past, SVCS was considered to be a medical emergency. However, multiple retrospective reviews have shown that this is not the case in the absence of laryngeal/bronchial or cerebral edema.[13,14,18] Accurate diagnosis via imaging and biopsy should be obtained, since treatment approaches can vary widely depending on the histology of the malignancy. Staging investigations should be completed before initiating treatment if possible, because a decision will need to be made regarding a definitive curative approach as opposed to a palliative course of treatment.

Although no standardized grading system exists for the evaluation of SVCS, the group from Yale University have recently proposed a classification system for grading the severity of SVCS[19] as asymptomatic (grade 0), mild (grade 1), moderate (grade 2), severe (grade 3), life-threatening (grade 4), or fatal (grade 5). Cerebral edema, laryngeal edema, stridor, and hemodynamic compromise would constitute grade 3 (if mild/moderate) or grade 4 (if significant) SVCS. The authors recommend more urgent treatment be initiated in the presence of grade 3 or 4 symptoms. The proposed system has not been validated but does provide a rational framework of how to approach and triage these patients.

The diagnosis of SVCS is made on the basis of clinical signs and symptoms and confirmed by imaging studies.

EVALUATION

Physical examination should document the extent of facial, neck, and/or arm swelling, elevation of neck veins, the extent of collateral veins on the chest, and any evidence of respiratory compromise. Facial swelling and plethora are typically exacerbated when patient is supine; the resultant cyanosis can be quite dramatic. Particular attention should be given to any palpable nodes, as they may provide an easily accessible site for tissue biopsy. Routine blood work should be obtained, including complete blood counts, renal function, and liver enzymes. Abnormalities in blood work may indicate other possible sites of biopsy, such as bone marrow or liver lesions, and may influence the subsequent therapy.

Imaging Studies

The majority of patients will have an abnormal chest radiograph (84%), with the most common findings being mediastinal widening (64%) and pleural effusion (26%).[12] **Fig. 1** is an example of a chest radiograph from a patient with SVCS. The most useful imaging study is computed tomography (CT) of the chest with contrast (needed to evaluate the SVC).[20,21] CT imaging allows the level and extent of the blockage to be defined as well as an evaluation of collateral pathways of drainage. It also permits identification of the cause of the obstruction, since a malignant mass is responsible for up to 90% of SVCS. Common findings on CT include enlarged paratracheal lymph nodes with or without additional lung or pleural abnormalities. A classic example of SVCS is shown in **Fig. 2**, where contrast clearly delineates compression of the SVC and the development of collateral vessels.

Venography is primarily used if an interventional stent is planned. Radionuclide Tc-99 m venography fails to provide the diagnostic information that is supplied by chest CT regarding location and characteristics of extrinsic masses. However, this technique can be useful for identifying thrombotic obstructions within the SVC.[22,23] Magnetic resonance imaging may be useful for patients who cannot tolerate CT contrast for any reason to assess mediastinal veins.[24,25]

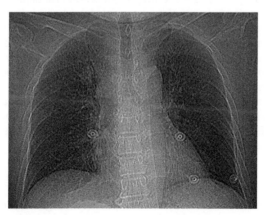

Fig. 1. Chest radiograph demonstrating mediastinal widening.

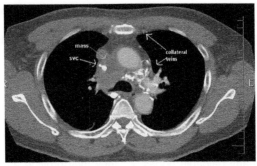

Fig. 2. Axial image of CT thorax, demonstrating a right paratracheal soft tissue mass causing narrowing and compression of SVC and presence of collaterals.

In addition to imaging of the chest, a full diagnostic workup for the suspected cancer may be appropriate either at this time or after the tissue diagnosis is obtained. For lung cancer, this typically includes imaging of the abdomen, brain, and bone; for lymphomas, this includes imaging of the abdomen and pelvis, possibly a bone marrow biopsy and a gallium and/or fluorodeoxyglucose positron emission tomographic scan, if appropriate.

Diagnostic Interventions

A tissue diagnosis is necessary to confirm the presence of a malignancy. In the absence of acute airway compromise or progressive neurologic decline from cerebral edema, initiation of therapy before obtaining a diagnosis is unwarranted given only infrequent reports of mortality from SVCS in multiple series.[13,14,18] However, the diagnostic workup should be expedited as patients may deteriorate quickly if collateral vessels are not well established. The importance of a proper diagnosis and staging of the patient cannot be overstressed. The treatment approaches vary widely depending on the type of malignancy present and whether an attempt will be made at definitive curative treatment as opposed to palliative approaches. Interventions such as radiation, chemotherapy, and/or steroids may obscure a histologic diagnosis at a later date. Radiation in particular can obscure a diagnosis in up to 42% of biopsy specimens obtained from the irradiated area after treatment.[26]

Careful clinical assessment of peripheral sites, such as supraclavicular nodes, that are easily accessible must be made before proceeding to more invasive procedures, such as bronchoscopy, mediastinoscopy, or endobronchial ultrasound guided biopsies (EBUS). Pleural effusions are also commonly found and are often accessible to thoracocentesis, although the diagnostic yield may be suboptimal.[27] Bronchoscopy has a diagnostic yield of 50% to 70% (depending on the presence of a centrally located lung mass), and transthoracic needle aspiration has a yield of 75%, whereas mediastinoscopy has a diagnostic yield of 90% to 100% in determining the cause of SVCS.[28–32] The risks associated with mediastinoscopy, predominantly bleeding and infection, are in the order of 0% to 7% in selected series.[28,29,31,33,34] No specific data exist with regard to the use of EBUS in obtaining a diagnosis in patients with SVCS, although randomized data suggest that EBUS is superior to conventional transbronchial needle aspiration in obtaining a diagnosis should mediastinoscopy be unavailable.[8,35]

MANAGEMENT

Management of superior cava syndrome due to malignancy depends on the etiology of the cancer, the extent of the disease, the severity of symptoms, and the prognosis of the patient.[19] Median life expectancy in patients with SVCS is approximately 6 months with a range of 1.5 to 9.5 months; however, estimates vary widely and are dependent on the underlying malignant condition.[36] Intervention needs to consider both treatment of the cancer and relief of the symptoms of the obstruction. Treatment of the cancer may be directed with curative intent or for palliation of symptoms alone. The intent of treatment is not always immediately clear, and therapy may need to be initiated before a full staging workup. For these reasons, the physician may wish to allow for a flexible treatment approach that would allow for conversion from a palliative approach to definitive management of the disease as the patient's status improves.

Data from randomized trials are scarce, and most evidence guiding treatment decisions are from case series. The treatment options include supportive measures, RT, chemotherapy, and stent insertion. Surgery is virtually never an option, as the presence of SVCS almost always signifies unresectable tumor within the mediastinum. Although there may be a role for surgery after induction treatment for selected patients with mediastinal nodal disease from lung cancer, it would be unlikely that a patient who presented with SVCS would have potentially resectable nodal disease. However, if in doubt, surgical input as part of multidisciplinary assessment may be sought, although the most efficient approach would be to refer to a specialist who is most likely to initiate appropriate therapy for the patient.

Interventions for Symptom Relief

Initial interventions should be directed toward supportive care and medical management. Although there are no data documenting the effectiveness of such maneuvers, these measures can be performed with minimal risk and may provide initial relief of the symptoms of SVCS. Oxygen support and attempts to minimize the hydrostatic pressure in the upper torso, such as fluid limitation, head elevation, and diuretics, may be useful in reducing symptoms in the short term.

Recognition of life-threatening symptoms suggestive of airway compromise and/or cerebral edema is essential. Evidence of severe airway compromise, such as stridor, accompanied by findings of laryngeal edema or tracheal obstruction on CT should be addressed emergently with interventions to protect the airway, such as an endotracheal tube. Management of cerebral edema associated with SVCS has not been described in the literature. Standard resuscitation techniques should be considered, such as head elevation, hyperventilation, and use of osmotic diuretics such as mannitol, if the patient presents with symptoms suggestive of cerebral edema. Imaging for an intracranial cause of cerebral edema should be obtained as well. In both cases, the patient should be hospitalized, monitored closely, and treated urgently to relieve the SVCS.

Steroids are often used as a temporary measure to reduce edema and associated symptoms,[37] but there is an absence of data documenting the effectiveness and dose of steroids in this setting. There is also a risk of obscuring the tissue diagnosis, especially if lymphoma is suspected.[3,5] In one retrospective review of 107 patients, the use of steroids and diuretics or neither therapy had a similar rate of clinical improvement of 84%.[13] However, in a symptomatic patient in whom airway edema is believed to contribute to the symptoms, steroids can be an effective intervention. No standard dosing or guidelines exist with regard to the dose of steroids to be used. At our institution, dexamethasone 4 mg orally twice a day or 4 mg orally four times a day is often initiated.

It should be emphasized that steroids should only be used as an initial temporizing measure. Chronic use of high doses of steroids can result in significant side effects, including facial swelling (cushingoid facies), and promote fluid retention, both of which could aggravate the symptoms of SVCS.[38,39] Prolonged use of high doses of cortico-steroids can also complicate assessment of therapeutic effectiveness, as the side effects of steroids can overlap with the symptoms of SVCS.

One should also be acutely aware that thrombosis may contribute to the severity of the SVCS as well as pose a major threat to life should pulmonary embolus or further thrombotic events occur. The incidence of thromboembolic events in patients with malignant SVCS has been reported as high as 38% in a group of prospectively followed patients.[40] There are less data guiding the decision to anticoagulate patients with malignant SVCS (without documented thrombus), with only an older, small, randomized trial that showed no difference in survival between patients anticoagulated versus those who were not.[41] Unfortunately, this trial did not report the incidence of pulmonary embolism. In summary, there is no evidence to support routine anticoagulation in patients with malignant SVCS in the absence of thrombosis. It appears reasonable to anticoagulate patients with demonstrable thrombus on imaging.

After a tissue diagnosis has been obtained and the extent of the disease has been determined, a decision should be made to address control of the malignant process in either a curative fashion or palliatively. Radiation, chemotherapy, or stent placement, or a combination of these modalities will play a role as the definitive intervention of SVCS, depending on the sensitivity of the specific tumor.

Radiation

Radiotherapy (RT) is an effective modality in the treatment of SVCS due to malignancy. A systemic review of the literature, conducted by Rowell and Gleeson,[5] documented that radiation was effective at providing overall relief in approximately three-quarters of SVCS due to SCLC and in two-thirds of SVCS due to non-small cell lung cancer (NSCLC).

The rapidity of response is in the range of 7 to 15 days but may be seen as early as 72 hours after initiation of therapy.[6,42–45] Relative contraindications to RT include previous treatment with radiation in the same region, certain connective tissue disorders such as scleroderma, and known radioresistant tumor types (eg, sarcoma). Response rates in the literature are often clinical, and there can be a significant discordance with objective response rates as measured by imaging. In one report, evaluation with serial venography documented complete relief in 31% and partial relief in 23% for a total objective response rate of 54%, which is somewhat lower than clinically reported response rates.[46]

The radiation treatment plan can vary based on the histology of the tumor as well as the intent of treatment. For example, a definitive course of radiation for SCLC can involve 3 to 6 weeks of daily or twice-a-day treatments (eg, 40 Gy in 15 daily fractions, 50 Gy in 25 fractions, 60 Gy in 30 fractions, or 45 Gy at fraction sizes of 1.5 Gy twice a day over 3 weeks). In NSCLC, definitive treatment takes 6 to 7 weeks to administer in daily fractions of 2 Gy. Palliative treatments are typically administered over a course of 1 to 2 weeks with larger fraction sizes of 3 Gy to 5 Gy (eg, 20 Gy in 5 fractions, 30 Gy in 10 fractions), with the goal of achieving a more rapid response by using larger daily doses. Abbreviated treatments of 2 6-Gy fractions (12 Gy/2 fractions) have been reported to be effective in older patients with poorer performance status.[47]

Radiation treatment planning usually involves CT-based simulation for designing RT fields. The fields should encompass the gross tumor volume and involved nodal regions and attempt to shield involved normal organs in the proximity of the tumor, particularly lung and esophagus, to minimize the risk of side effects. The size and configuration of the fields may be altered during the treatment course, as patients may improve symptomatically, and tumor may shrink to allow for a higher curative dose to be delivered.

Careful assessment of the patient is needed during the radiation treatment to monitor for side effects as well as progression of radioresistant tumors necessitating alternative interventions, such as stent placement and/or a protective airway if symptoms worsen. Occasionally, worsening of symptoms can be due to development of a thrombus, in which case vascular imaging and anticoagulation should be considered.

Chemotherapy

Lymphomas, SCLCs, and germ cell tumors are widely regarded as chemotherapy-sensitive tumors, with high rates of response and quick onset of tumor shrinkage. Thus, chemotherapy is often used as the initial treatment for SVCS from such tumors. RT alone can be used and can provide prompt responses as well for these malignancies; but it usually yields poorer long-term results and is used only in patients who are not candidates for chemotherapy.[4,6] Chemotherapy can relieve the symptoms of SVCS in up to 80% of patients with NHL and 77% with SCLS.[4,5] The response rate of relief from SVCS treated with chemotherapy is similar to that of RT and ranges from 7 to 15 days.[36] **Fig. 3** demonstrates the response of a patient with a chemotherapy-sensitive tumor. After several cycles of chemotherapy, the patient recovered patency of his SVC with good symptomatic relief and reduction in tumor burden.

The addition of RT to chemotherapy did not significantly affect the relief of SVCS or relapse rates in 2 randomized trials of SCLC and NSCLC as well as in a systemic review of the published data.[5,8,48] Once the symptomatic benefit is obtained, the patient may be a candidate for curative treatment, which in cases of limited-stage SCLC or early stage NHL would include the addition of RT to systemic chemotherapy, as this has been shown to decrease local recurrence rates and improve survival in these clinical scenarios.

Endovascular Stenting

Endovascular stenting can provide rapid relief by restoring venous return in patients with SVCS. Relief can be immediate, but in most series, it is reported within 24 to 72 hours following the procedure.[5,49–51] Stent placement can be especially useful when urgent intervention is indicated for patients without a tissue diagnosis or who have previously been treated with RT or in those who have known chemotherapy- and radiation-resistant tumors. In addition, endovascular stenting may be considered as a first-line intervention in patients with SVCS.[52–54] Stents provide relief from the

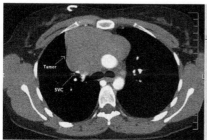
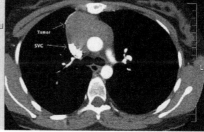

Prechemotherapy   2 months post-chemotherapy

Fig. 3. Radiographic response of patient with malignant SVCS from a chemotherapy-sensitive tumor.

obstruction in an immediate and direct fashion, but they do not deal with the cancer itself. Thus, in many cases, stent placement is followed by other treatments, such as radiation and/or chemotherapy.

Stent placement is usually performed under local anesthesia in an angiography suite, with introduction of a guide wire via either the subclavian or internal jugular vein with or without balloon angioplasty followed by deployment of a stent.[53,55,56] If a clot is encountered, thrombolytics are often used, although their benefit in this context remains unclear, and the morbidity of stent placement does appear higher with the use of thrombolytics.[32,36,57] Even in the absence of a visible thrombus, some advocate use of prophylactic anticoagulation (eg, with low-molecular-weight heparin) after stent placement, given the presence of a foreign body and the fact that cancer patients (particularly lung cancer patients) are at an increased risk of thrombosis. Whether this is clearly beneficial is not known. The use of steroids is also not mentioned in most studies.[36] Whether or not a particular type of stent is advantageous remains unknown.[58,59]

There are no randomized, controlled trials comparing the efficacy of endovascular stenting with radiation or chemotherapy. The most extensive data come from a systemic review of the literature by Rowell and Gleeson in which 23 stent studies were combined for a total of 159 patients with SVCS due to either SCLC or NSCLC.[36] The results were not reported separately for the different histologies. About 95% of the patients experienced complete or partial relief of their symptoms following stenting; the relapse rate was reported as 11%. In comparison, relief rates in 487 patients with SCLC treated with chemotherapy alone, chemoradiotherapy, or RT were 77%, 83%, and 78% respectively; however, in NSCLC, relief rates in 243 patients treated with chemotherapy or RT were 59% and 63%, respectively.[36] From this review, stenting appears to be the most effective and rapid treatment available to patients with SVCS due to malignancy. However, there are far fewer patients treated with stents in the literature, and patient selection may have played a role. Thus, comparison of outcomes is limited due to the absence of randomized studies. Obtaining randomized data for a direct comparison is difficult for a number of reasons: one treatment may be more immediately available than the other (eg, there may not be stent expertise, or radiation may not be immediately available), or there may be a clinical reason to favor one over the other (eg, stent may be preferred in a previous irradiated chest area; radiation can be initiated quickly if there are also symptoms of airway compromise; chemotherapy may be chosen if it is a chemosensitive tumor).[60] Thus, although randomized trials have been attempted, to date, they have not been successfully completed.[60] Whether endovascular stenting is truly superior in longer-term palliation of the symptoms of SVCS remains unknown.

SUMMARY AND RECOMMENDATIONS

SVCS is a common complication of malignancies such as lung cancer or lymphoma. The presentation is often clinically striking, especially if not recognized early enough. It requires a workup and formulation of a management plan, although not necessarily an emergency intervention. In most cases, the initial management of this syndrome should be directed at supportive care, including such maneuvers as elevation of the head, oxygen support, diuretics, and possibly steroids, although none has been proven to be of benefit. This should be followed by confirmation of the presence of venous obstruction with imaging and interventions to establish the etiology. A histologic diagnosis confirming malignancy should be obtained before initiating therapy in a patient with no previous diagnosis of cancer. Steroids are often used to decrease

Table 1
Advantages and disadvantages of radiation therapy, stent insertion, and chemotherapy

Radiation		Stent		Chemotherapy	
Advantages	*Disadvantages*	*Advantages*	*Disadvantages*	*Advantages*	*Disadvantages*
Noninvasive intervention	Symptom relief in 7–15 d	Rapid relief of symptoms usually within 24–72 h	Invasive intervention	Noninvasive intervention	Symptom relief in 7–15 d
Treats underlying malignancy	May compromise a tissue diagnosis if not yet obtained	Does not compromise a tissue diagnosis	Bleeding complications	Treats underlying malignancy	May compromise a tissue diagnosis if not yet obtained
—	May initially worsen symptoms due to inflammation	Allows option for further treatment with chemotherapy, radiation, or combined-modality therapy	Increased risk of thrombosis due to foreign object	Does not require specialized equipment	Patient may be too sick to tolerate chemotherapy
—	—	—	Does not treat the underlying malignancy	Ability to be administered in ICU	Hematologic and other toxicity

Abbreviation: ICU, intensive care unit.
The interventions are supported by level of evidence B; there is no level A evidence specific to the management of SVCS.

swelling but may obscure a histologic diagnosis. In patients with life-threatening signs, such as worsening laryngeal edema and stridorous symptoms, initial placement of an intravascular stent can provide rapid relief without compromising future treatments or diagnostic interventions. One should also be vigilant for the presence or development of thrombosis in these patients. There are no data to support routine anticoagulation in patients with malignant SVCS without evidence of thrombus.

Following a diagnosis of malignancy, a decision should be made as to whether the intent of treatment will be curative or palliative. Treatment planning should be multidisciplinary and include medical and radiation oncologists at an early stage. Treatment options include stent placement, radiation alone, chemotherapy alone, and combined-modality therapy. No randomized studies have shown superiority of one approach over the other, and the choice should be tailored to the particular clinical scenario.

For patients with a newly diagnosed chemotherapy- sensitive malignancy, such as SCLC, NHL, and germ cell tumors, systemic chemotherapy as an initial intervention is reasonable. The use of stents in severely symptomatic patients can provide rapid relief if necessary. Radiation alone is also an effective intervention in these malignancies should chemotherapy be unavailable or contraindicated.

For patients with a newly diagnosed NSCLC, endovascular stent placement or RT is recommended as a first intervention. RT may be used alone or as part of a combined-modality approach with concurrent or sequential chemotherapy. A direct comparison of RT and stent placement has not been made in a randomized, control setting, but it appears from retrospective reports that stent placement is at least as effective as radiation with regard to relief rates and is certainly more rapid. A qualitative comparison of the 3 interventions is presented in **Table 1**.

For patients who have recurrent or progressive malignancies and symptomatic SVC who have had previous radiation in the mediastinum, we recommend consideration of endovascular stents for relief of symptoms. Whether or not radiation can be delivered to the same area again will depend on the dose and technique of previous radiation. If previous RT was administered with palliative intent, ie, lower to moderate doses, further RT may be possible, but would require careful planning to avoid organs at risk of re-irradiation, particularly the spinal cord, if treated before. If previous RT was high dose, it may not be possible to safely deliver further RT, and stent would indeed be the best consideration.

For patients who are treated with radiation with severe airway obstruction, a short course of steroids (dexamethasone 4 mg orally twice a day to 4 mg orally four times a day) is reasonable during the radiation to prevent further compromise due to worsening swelling caused by acute radiation response, but there is no evidence supporting this intervention.

The treatment of SVCS secondary to malignancy must be individualized, based on previous treatments as well as overall prognosis. The median survival in patients presenting with SVCS ranges from 1.5 to 9.5 months in the literature and must be kept in mind when tailoring an approach for these patients.[5] For patients with short life expectancy, the focus will be on short-term symptom relief. For patients with longer prognosis, more definitive treatment targeting not only the obstruction but the local tumors would provide better chances of control of SVCS.

REFERENCES

1. Armstrong BA, Perez CA, Simpson JR, et al. Role of irradiation in the management of superior vena cava syndrome. Int J Radiat Oncol Biol Phys 1987;13(4): 531–9.

2. Markman M. Diagnosis and management of superior vena cava syndrome. Cleve Clin J Med 1999;66(1):59–61.
3. Ostler PJ, Clarke DP, Watkinson AF, et al. Superior vena cava obstruction: a modern management strategy. Clin Oncol (R Coll Radiol) 1997;9(2):83–9.
4. Perez-Soler R, McLaughlin P, Velasquez WS, et al. Clinical features and results of management of superior vena cava syndrome secondary to lymphoma. J Clin Oncol 1984;2(4):260–6.
5. Rowell NP, Gleeson FV. Steroids, radiotherapy, chemotherapy and stents for superior vena caval obstruction in carcinoma of the bronchus: a systematic review. Clin Oncol (R Coll Radiol) 2002;14(5):338–51.
6. Sculier JP, Evans WK, Feld R, et al. Superior vena caval obstruction syndrome in small cell lung cancer. Cancer 1986;57(4):847–51.
7. Chen YM, Yang S, Perng RP, et al. Superior vena cava syndrome revisited. Jpn J Clin Oncol 1995;25(2):32–6.
8. Spiro SG, Shah S, Harper PG, et al. Treatment of obstruction of the superior vena cava by combination chemotherapy with and without irradiation in small-cell carcinoma of the bronchus. Thorax 1983;38(7):501–5.
9. Presswala RG, Hiranandani NL. Pleural effusion and superior vena cava canal syndrome in Hodgkin's disease. J Indian Med Assoc 1965;45(9):502–3.
10. Lazzarino M, Orlandi E, Paulli M, et al. Primary mediastinal B-cell lymphoma with sclerosis: an aggressive tumor with distinctive clinical and pathologic features. J Clin Oncol 1993;11(12):2306–13.
11. Rice TW, Rodriguez RM, Light RW. The superior vena cava syndrome: clinical characteristics and evolving etiology. Medicine (Baltimore) 2006;85(1):37–42.
12. Parish JM, Marschke RF Jr, Dines DE, et al. Etiologic considerations in superior vena cava syndrome. Mayo Clin Proc 1981;56(7):407–13.
13. Schraufnagel DE, Hill R, Leech JA, et al. Superior vena caval obstruction. Is it a medical emergency? Am J Med 1981;70(6):1169–74.
14. Yellin A, Rosen A, Reichert N, et al. Superior vena cava syndrome. The myth–the facts. Am Rev Respir Dis 1990;141(5 Pt 1):1114–8.
15. Eren S, Karaman A, Okur A. The superior vena cava syndrome caused by malignant disease. Imaging with multi-detector row CT. Eur J Radiol 2006;59(1):93–103.
16. Stanford W, Jolles H, Ell S, et al. Superior vena cava obstruction: a venographic classification. AJR Am J Roentgenol 1987;148(2):259–62.
17. Kim HJ, Kim HS, Chung SH. CT diagnosis of superior vena cava syndrome: importance of collateral vessels. AJR Am J Roentgenol 1993;161(3):539–42.
18. Gauden SJ. Superior vena cava syndrome induced by bronchogenic carcinoma: is this an oncological emergency? Australas Radiol 1993;37(4):363–6.
19. Yu JB, Wilson LD, Detterbeck FC. Superior vena cava syndrome–a proposed classification system and algorithm for management. J Thorac Oncol 2008; 3(8):811–4.
20. Schwartz EE, Goodman LR, Haskin ME. Role of CT scanning in the superior vena cava syndrome. Am J Clin Oncol 1986;9(1):71–8.
21. Bechtold RE, Wolfman NT, Karstaedt N, et al. Superior vena caval obstruction: detection using CT. Radiology 1985;157(2):485–7.
22. Conte FA, Orzel JA. Superior vena cava syndrome and bilateral subclavian vein thrombosis. CT and radionuclide venography correlation. Clin Nucl Med 1986; 11(10):698–700.
23. Podoloff DA, Kim EE. Evaluation of sensitivity and specificity of upper extremity radionuclide venography in cancer patients with indwelling central venous catheters. Clin Nucl Med 1992;17(6):457–62.

24. Hansen ME, Spritzer CE, Sostman HD. Assessing the patency of mediastinal and thoracic inlet veins: value of MR imaging. AJR Am J Roentgenol 1990;155(6): 1177–82.
25. Hartnell GG, Hughes LA, Finn JP, et al. Magnetic resonance angiography of the central chest veins. A new gold standard? Chest 1995;107(4):1053–7.
26. Loeffler JS, Leopold KA, Recht A, et al. Emergency prebiopsy radiation for mediastinal masses: impact on subsequent pathologic diagnosis and outcome. J Clin Oncol 1986;4(5):716–21.
27. Rice TW, Rodriquez RM, Barnette R, et al. Prevalence and characteristics of pleural effusions in superior vena cava syndrome. Respirology 2006;11(3):299–305.
28. Mineo TC, Ambrogi V, Nofroni I, et al. Mediastinoscopy in superior vena cava obstruction: analysis of 80 consecutive patients. Ann Thorac Surg 1999;68(1): 223–6.
29. Porte H, Metois D, Finzi L, et al. Superior vena cava syndrome of malignant origin. Which surgical procedure for which diagnosis? Eur J Cardiothorac Surg 2000; 17(4):384–8.
30. Selcuk ZT, Firat P. The diagnostic yield of transbronchial needle aspiration in superior vena cava syndrome. Lung Cancer 2003;42(2):183–8.
31. Trinkle JK, Bryant I R, Malette WG, et al. Mediastinoscopy–diagnostic value compared to bronchoscopy: scalene biopsy and sputum cytology in 155 patients. Am Surg 1968;34(10):740–3.
32. Wilson LD, Detterbeck FC, Yahalom J. Clinical practice. Superior vena cava syndrome with malignant causes. N Engl J Med 2007;356(18):1862–9.
33. Jahangiri M, Taggart DP, Goldstraw P. Role of mediastinoscopy in superior vena cava obstruction. Cancer 1993;71(10):3006–8.
34. Callejas MA, Rami R, Catalan M, et al. Mediastinoscopy as an emergency diagnostic procedure in superior vena cava syndrome. Scand J Thorac Cardiovasc Surg 1991;25(2):137–9.
35. Herth F, Becker HD, Ernst A. Conventional vs endobronchial ultrasound-guided transbronchial needle aspiration: a randomized trial. Chest 2004;125(1):322–5.
36. Rowell NP, Gleeson FV. Steroids, radiotherapy, chemotherapy and stents for superior vena caval obstruction in carcinoma of the bronchus. Cochrane Database Syst Rev 2001;(4):CD001316.
37. Kaplan AP, Greaves MW. Angioedema. J Am Acad Dermatol 2005;53(3):373–88, quiz 389–92.
38. McDougall R, Sibley J, Haga M, et al. Outcome in patients with rheumatoid arthritis receiving prednisone compared to matched controls. J Rheumatol 1994;21(7):1207–13.
39. Wei L, MacDonald TM, Walker BR. Taking glucocorticoids by prescription is associated with subsequent cardiovascular disease. Ann Intern Med 2004;141(10):764–70.
40. Adelstein DJ, Hines JD, Carter SG, et al. Thromboembolic events in patients with malignant superior vena cava syndrome and the role of anticoagulation. Cancer 1988;62(10):2258–62.
41. Ghosh BC, Cliffton EE. Malignant tumors with superior vena cava obstruction. N Y State J Med 1973;73(2):283–9.
42. Dombernowsky P, Hansen HH. Combination chemotherapy in the management of superior vena caval obstruction in small-cell anaplastic carcinoma of the lung. Acta Med Scand 1978;204(6):513–6.
43. Kane RC, Cohen MH. Superior vena caval obstruction due to small-cell anaplastic lung carcinoma. Response to chemotherapy. JAMA 1976;235(16): 1717–8.

44. Maddox AM, Valdivieso M, Lukeman J, et al. Superior vena cava obstruction in small cell bronchogenic carcinoma. Clinical parameters and survival. Cancer 1983;52(11):2165–72.
45. Tan EH, Ang PT. Resolution of superior vena cava obstruction in small cell lung cancer patients treated with chemotherapy. Ann Acad Med Singap 1995;24(6): 812–5.
46. Ahmann FR. A reassessment of the clinical implications of the superior vena caval syndrome. J Clin Oncol 1984;2(8):961–9.
47. Lonardi F, Gioga G, Graziella A, et al. Double-flash, large-fraction radiation therapy as palliative treatment of malignant superior vena cava syndrome in the elderly. Support Care Cancer 2002;10(2):156–60.
48. Pereira JR, Martins CJ, Ikari FK, et al. Neoadjuvant chemotherapy vs. radio-therapy alone for superior vena cava syndrome (SVCS) due to non-small cell lung cancer (NSCLC): preliminary results of a randomized phase II trial. Eur J Cancer 1999;35(Suppl 4):260.
49. Hennequin LM, Fade O, Fays JG, et al. Superior vena cava stent placement: results with the Wallstent endoprosthesis. Radiology 1995;196(2):353–61.
50. Irving JD, Dondelinger RF, Reidy JF, et al. Gianturco self-expanding stents: clin-ical experience in the vena cava and large veins. Cardiovasc Intervent Radiol 1992;15(5):328–33.
51. Rosch J, Uchida BT, Hall LD, et al. Gianturco-Rosch expandable Z-stents in the treatment of superior vena cava syndrome. Cardiovasc Intervent Radiol 1992; 15(5):319–27.
52. Bierdrager E, Lampmann LE, Lohle PN, et al. Endovascular stenting in neoplastic superior vena cava syndrome prior to chemotherapy or radiotherapy. Neth J Med 2005;63(1):20–3.
53. Greillier L, Barlesi F, Doddoli C, et al. Vascular stenting for palliation of superior vena cava obstruction in non-small-cell lung cancer patients: a future 'standard' procedure? Respiration 2004;71(2):178–83.
54. Kim YI, Kim KS, Ko YC, et al. Endovascular stenting as a first choice for the palli-ation of superior vena cava syndrome. J Korean Med Sci 2004;19(4):519–22.
55. de Gregorio Ariza MA, Gamboa P, Gimeno MJ, et al. Percutaneous treatment of superior vena cava syndrome using metallic stents. Eur Radiol 2003;13(4): 853–62.
56. Nagata T, Makutani S, Uchida H, et al. Follow-up results of 71 patients under-going metallic stent placement for the treatment of a malignant obstruction of the superior vena cava. Cardiovasc Intervent Radiol 2007;30(5):959–67.
57. Crowe MT, Davies CH, Gaines PA. Percutaneous management of superior vena cava occlusions. Cardiovasc Intervent Radiol 1995;18(6):367–72.
58. Oudkerk M, Kuijpers TJ, Schmitz PI, et al. Self-expanding metal stents for pallia-tive treatment of superior vena caval syndrome. Cardiovasc Intervent Radiol 1996;19(3):146–51.
59. Schindler N, Vogelzang RL. Superior vena cava syndrome. Experience with endovascular stents and surgical therapy. Surg Clin North Am 1999;79(3): 683–94, xi.
60. Wilson P, Bezjak A, Asch M, et al. The difficulties of a randomized study in supe-rior vena caval obstruction. J Thorac Oncol 2007;2(6):514–9.

Cerebral Edema, Altered Mental Status, Seizures, Acute Stroke, Leptomeningeal Metastases, and Paraneoplastic Syndrome

Denise M. Damek, MD[a,b,c,*]

KEYWORDS

- Cerebral edema • Altered mental status
- Seizures • Acute stroke • Leptomeningeal metastases
- Paraneoplastic syndrome

Neurologic disorders are a frequent cause of emergency department (ED) visits, subspecialty consultation, and hospital admissions in oncology patients.[1–3] Neurologic disorders are often the presenting symptom of systemic cancer. In addition, neurologic complications are a source of significant disability, morbidity, and mortality in cancer patients. This article provides an overview of selected cancer-related neurologic emergencies that present to the ED, including cerebral edema and increased intracranial pressure, altered mental status, seizures, acute stroke, leptomeningeal metastases, and paraneoplastic neurologic syndromes.

A version of this article was previously published in the *Emergency Medicine Clinics of North America*, 27:2.

[a] Neuro-Oncology, University of Colorado Denver School of Medicine, 12631 East 17th Avenue, MS# B-185, Aurora, CO 80045, USA

[b] Department of Neurology, University of Colorado Denver School of Medicine, 12631 East 17th Avenue, MS# B-185, Aurora, CO 80045, USA

[c] Department of Neurosurgery, University of Colorado Denver School of Medicine, 12631 East 17th Avenue, MS# B-185, Aurora, CO 80045, USA

* Neuro-Oncology, University of Colorado Denver School of Medicine, 12631 East 17th Avenue, MS# B-185, Aurora, CO 80045.

E-mail address: denise.damek@ucdenver.edu

Hematol Oncol Clin N Am 24 (2010) 515–535
doi:10.1016/j.hoc.2010.03.010
0889-8588/10/$ – see front matter © 2010 Elsevier Inc. All rights reserved.

CEREBRAL EDEMA AND INCREASED INTRACRANIAL PRESSURE

As a brain tumor enlarges, it produces focal findings by invasion and compression of surrounding brain tissue. More generalized signs and symptoms, such as headache, nausea, vomiting, papilledema, and depressed levels of consciousness, result from increased intracranial pressure due to the space occupied by the tumor mass, associated cerebral edema, or obstruction of cerebrospinal fluid outflow pathways.

Vasogenic edema occurs as tumor growth leads to disruption of the blood-brain barrier and increased capillary permeability, which allows a protein- and sodium-rich plasma filtrate to enter the extracellular fluid space and spread throughout adjacent white matter. Increased hydrostatic pressure within the tumor, an osmotic gradient, and the absence of a lymphatic system within the central nervous system also lead to extracellular fluid accumulation. As a result, focal mass effect, increased intracranial pressure, compromise of local blood supply, or brain herniation syndromes may occur.

Headaches are reported at presentation by approximately one half of all brain tumor patients, especially those with rapidly growing neoplasms or infratentorial tumors. At first glance these headaches may seem nondescript, but there are characteristics of headache in this patient population that the ED triage team will find valuable. Brain tumor patients generally describe a dull nonthrobbing headache similar to a tension headache. The headache is mild at onset, becoming increasingly more severe over days and weeks, and is typically associated with other symptoms of increased intracranial pressure and focal neurologic deficits. In fact, less than 10% of brain tumor patients have isolated headache syndromes, making the presence of abnormal neurologic signs and symptoms an important diagnostic distinction between tumor-related and benign headaches.[4] The classic brain tumor headache syndrome, characterized as a dull, aching pain that awakens the patient from sleep or is present on awakening with improvement thereafter, and often aggravated by positional change or Valsalva maneuvers, or associated with nausea and vomiting, is actually rare to nonexistent. Obstructive hydrocephalus is often associated with a more acute headache presentation and vomiting.

Patients with brain tumors may also experience headaches in conjunction with plateau pressure waves. Under normal circumstances, vasomotor tone automatically adjusts to maintain constant intracranial pressure with positional changes or other variables. However, in patients with brain tumors, mass effect and other factors can impede vasomotor autoregulation leading to plateau pressure waves that are characterized by the abrupt rapid elevation of intracranial pressure for brief 5- to 20-minute periods.[5] This sudden change in intracranial pressure produces short duration (20–30 minutes) headaches that are precipitated by a change in posture, and are often accompanied by an abrupt decline in mental status and emesis. Level of alertness is generally unaffected, but loss of consciousness can occur. These symptoms may be confused with seizure activity in patients with a known diagnosis of brain tumor.

Altered mental status is the initial symptom or sign in one third of brain tumor patients. Disturbances range from psychomotor retardation to lethargy to obtundation and coma. Papilledema is noted in approximately 8% of malignant glioma patients at presentation.[4] Most patients with papilledema do not report ocular symptoms, but some report transient visual obscurations or blurred vision. Visual acuity is generally unaffected. Early fundoscopic manifestations of papilledema include disc hyperemia, subtle edema of the nasal disc, small hemorrhages of the nerve fiber layer, and loss of spontaneous venous pulsations, which are normally present in 80% of the population. Later, the disc becomes grossly elevated, the margins obscure, and hemorrhage, exudates, and cotton wool spots may occur. Increased intracranial pressure may also cause vomiting, with or without nausea, as pressure is exerted on brain stem structures. Vague nonvertiginous dizziness is a frequent accompaniment. Projectile vomiting without nausea frequently occurs in patients with posterior fossa tumors and obstructive hydrocephalus.

Focal mass lesions can result in the asymmetric shift of brain contents from one intracranial compartment to another, producing herniation syndromes (**Table 1**). False localizing signs are more commonly seen with slow growing neoplasms that produce prolonged elevation of intracranial pressure and chronic tissue shift.[6] Acute herniation syndromes involving the medial temporal lobes (transtentorial herniation) or the cerebellar tonsils (tonsillar herniation), are often fatal and treatment outcomes, when successful, are poor. The earliest manifestation of transtentorial herniation is unilateral papillary dilatation and decrease in level of consciousness followed by ipsilateral or contralateral hemiparesis. Tonsillar herniation leads to compression of the respiratory centers in the medulla and ultimately respiratory arrest. Careful observation during recording of vital signs by the ED triage team may allow for the appreciation of warning signs of impending herniation such as abnormal breathing patterns (Cheyne-Stokes, central neurogenic hyperventilation, Biot's breathing), repetitive respiratory reflexes (sighing, yawning, hiccups), and Cushing's triad, which consists of bradycardia, hypertension, and change in respiratory pattern.

Currently there is no standard protocol or algorithm to guide the emergency medicine physician for the management of increased intracranial pressure or brain herniation. Likewise, there is a paucity of prospective clinical trial data on which to base management. General treatment approaches are contingent on rapidity and severity of neurologic symptoms, and vary widely from institution to institution. In some cases, medical management may reverse herniation syndromes, or serve to temporarily stabilize the patient until surgical decompression is possible.

Corticosteroids

Glucocorticoids, in particular dexamethasone, play a major role in the management of symptomatic cerebral edema.[7,8] Approximately 70% to 80% of brain tumor patients will experience symptom improvement following dexamethasone treatment.[9] In nonemergent clinical situations, the daily dose of dexamethasone ranges from 6 mg to 24 mg and is typically divided into 2 to 4 doses.[7] The long half-life of dexamethasone permits twice daily dosing, and the provision of 4 daily doses has become entrenched in current medical practice. In patients with impaired consciousness, rapidly progressing signs of increased intracranial pressure, or cerebral herniation, an intravenous bolus of dexamethasone (40–100 mg) followed by a maintenance dose of dexamethasone of 40 to 100 mg over 24 hours in divided doses may be effective in reversing symptoms. Concurrent provision of 20 mg of intravenous furosemide may further augment the effect of the steroid.

Physiologically, the first change after steroid administration is a decrease in plateau waves followed by a gradual decline in intracranial pressure over 48 to 72 hours.[10] Symptomatic improvement can be seen within the first few hours of intravenous steroid therapy, and maximal clinical improvement is generally achieved within 24 to 72 hours. Evidence of generalized brain dysfunction typically improves before focal neurologic symptoms or signs. If the desired clinical response is not achieved within 48 hours of standard dexamethasone dosing, the dose can be doubled every 48 hours until clinical response or a total daily dose of 100 mg of dexamethasone is

Table 1
Brain herniation syndromes

Type of Herniation	Definition	Symptoms/Signs
Transtentorial herniation		
• Descending	Downward displacement of the brain through the tentorium at the level of the incisura	• Compression of ipsilateral cranial nerve III may lead to dilatation of the pupil and extraocular eye movement abnormalities • Compression of ipsilateral corticospinal tracts cause contralateral hemiparesis • Compression of the posterior cerebral artery may cause unilateral or bilateral occipital lobe infarction • Compression of the pontine perforating vessels may cause brain stem hemorrhage • Compression of the midbrain may cause hydrocephalus • Kernohan notch phenomenon is caused by compression of the contralateral cerebral peduncle against the adjacent tentorium causing false, localizing ipsilateral hemiparesis
• Ascending	Upward displacement of brain through the tentorium at the level of the incisura	• Depending on rapidity of shift, brain stem compression may cause nausea or vomiting, hycrocephalus, or rapid progression to coma
Subfalcine/cingulated herniation	Displacement of brain underneath the falx	• May be asymptomatic • Headache • Contralateral leg weakness • Compression of the anterior cerebral artery may cause ipsilateral frontal lobe infarction
Tonsillar herniation	Downward displacement of infratentorial brain through the foramen magnum	• Acute compression of the brain stem may cause obtundation, rapidly progressing to death • Insidious processes may cause Lhermitte phenomenon
Sphenoid/alar herniation	Supratentorial brain displaced anteriorly or posteriorly over the wing of the sphenoid bone	Frequently asymptomatic
• Anterior	Temporal lobe displaced anteriorly and superiorly over the sphenoid bone	—
• Posterior	Frontal lobe is displaced posteriorly and inferiorly over the sphenoid bone	—
Extracranial herniation	Displacement of brain through a cranial defect	Herniated brain may become ischemic

reached.[11,12] The patient should then be maintained on the lowest dose necessary to maintain symptom control.

Hyperventilation

Intubation and hyperventilation to a target partial pressure of carbon dioxide (pCO_2) of 30 mm Hg remains the most rapid means of decreasing increased intracranial pressure. As the pCO_2 decreases, cerebral vasoconstriction in undamaged areas of the brain occurs, resulting in decreased cerebral blood volume and intracranial pressure. The benefit of hyperventilation manifests within 30 seconds and is maintained for about 15 to 20 minutes.[13] Thereafter, a compensatory metabolic acidosis negates its effect. The primary usefulness of hyperventilation is to gain immediate control of intracranial pressure, allowing time for other treatment modalities to take effect.

Osmotherapy

Hyperosmolar agents create an osmotic gradient that effectively draws water from the extracellular space to the higher osmolarity in blood, thereby reducing brain volume and intracranial pressure. Historically, mannitol is the most commonly used osmotic agent; however, there is growing evidence in support of the use of hypertonic saline.[14,15] Mannitol is typically provided as a 20% to 25% solution and given as a 0.5- to 2.0-g/kg intravenous loading dose. The effect of mannitol manifests within 15 to 30 minutes and is generally sustained for several hours.[13,16] If clinically warranted repeated small intravenous boluses may be administered, however, repeated doses of mannitol may precipitate rebound intracranial hypertension. The provision of a loop diuretic such as furosemide given 15 to 20 minutes after mannitol as a one time 20-mg intravenous dose may augment the benefit of mannitol.[17] Hypertonic saline at concentrations ranging from 3% to 23.4% seems to be as effective if not superior to mannitol with a more favorable side effect profile.[15,18–20] However, unlike mannitol, hypertonic saline is a significant vesicant, which should be preferentially infused into a central line.

Adjunct Therapies

Additional adjuncts to the management of increased intracranial pressure and acute herniation syndromes include elevation of the head, propofol or pentobarbital anesthesia, and hypothermia. Elevation of the head by 30 degrees with care to avoid flexion or extension of the neck maximizes venous outflow. Propofol induces vasoconstriction and decreases the cerebral metabolic rate of oxygen, which in turn reduces cerebral blood flow, cerebral blood volume, and intracranial pressure.[21] Barbiturates also suppress cerebral metabolism, which subsequently decreases cerebral blood flow and cerebral blood volumes. Hypothermia can reduce the cerebral metabolism rate of oxygen by 5% per degree reduction in core body temperature, thereby decreasing cerebral blood flow and intracranial pressure. However, increased risk of cardiac dysrhythmias, coagulopathy, and systemic infection limit its usefulness.

ALTERED MENTAL STATUS
Delirium

Delirium occurs in 25% to 40% of patients with cancer, and is present in up to 90% of terminally ill cancer patients.[22] Delirium, often used synonymously with acute confusion, is the most common cause of neurologic consultation in cancer patients, and results in upwards of 10% of admissions to general oncology wards.[2,22–24] The syndrome is characterized by rapid onset over hours or days of fluctuating abnormalities of thought, perception, and levels of awareness. More specifically, decreased attention and disorganized thinking are accompanied by variable altered level of consciousness, disorientation, decreased short term memory, hallucinations or illusions, alteration of sleep-wake cycle, and abnormal behavior modulation. Mood and behavior changes are often the primary outward manifestation of delirium. Patients may exhibit loud, boisterous, aggressive, and agitated behavior, or alternatively may have quiet, reserved, and passive behavior, and appear depressed. Brief simplistic psychotic ideas are commonly present, and neurologic signs such as unsteady gait and tremor may be seen.

Delirium often goes unrecognized, or may be confused with dementia, depression, psychoses, seizures, or attributed erroneously to terminal illness. In addition, it is consistently associated with more numerous and longer hospital stays, and increased morbidity and mortality.[24]

Delirium remains a clinical diagnosis. Although various instruments or assessment tools have been developed to screen patients for delirium, they remain largely unvalidated, unstudied, and unused in patients with cancer.[25] Key to recognition of delirium is a clear understanding of the patient's baseline cognitive functioning, as well as critical assessment of ongoing symptoms, which may require ancillary history from family members or other caregivers. In addition, a high index of suspicion, and awareness of associated risk factors and etiologies of delirium in the cancer patient is required of the ED team.

Delirium may result from direct and indirect effects of cancer and its treatment on the central nervous system. Multiple precipitating factors were identified in more than 60% of cancer patients with delirium, with a median number of 3 probable causes per patient.[22–24] The most common causes of delirium in the cancer patient included drugs, systemic infection, structural brain lesions, and metabolic dysfunction.[23,24] Metabolic aberrations included hyponatremia, hypoxia or hypoperfusion, and renal failure.[24] Cancer type and chemotherapy were not generally contributing factors.[24] In one report, low albumin levels were found in 80% of patients, but cachexia was not recorded and the extent of malnutrition was not known.[24] Similar to reports in noncancer patients, surgical procedures precipitated delirium in up to 40% of patients.[24,26] Likewise, infection was a strong risk factor for delirium, but it rarely occurred in isolation.[23,24] Data from elderly, noncancer patients found that delirium, not an elevated temperature, was frequently the first sign of sepsis.[27,28] Nonconvulsive status epilepticus (NCSE) may be an under-recognized cause of delirium in comatose patients.[29,30]

It is critical that the emergency medicine physician appreciates that delirium is reversible with appropriate intervention in more than 50% of patients.[22,24] Moreover, meaningful functional improvement can be seen in patients with advanced cancer if any reversible contributing factors are treated. Reversible precipitants of delirium include opioid and nonopioid psychoactive medications, dehydration, infection, surgical procedures, structural brain abnormalities, and NCSE.[22–24,29,31–33] Rapid improvement is frequently seen in patients with brain tumors or hemorrhagic metastases after administration of corticosteroids, which is often initiated in the ED.[24]

With few exceptions, the diagnostic evaluation of delirium in cancer patients does not differ from that routinely undertaken in noncancer patients. Neuroimaging is indicated in most cancer patients with delirium including those with a nonfocal examination, the exception being patients who rapidly clear following a medical intervention. Notably, lateralizing signs are absent in one fourth of patients with delirium and a structural brain lesion on neuroimaging.[24] Electroencephalography is indicated in comatose or significantly clouded patients; the reported incidence of NCSE in these patients is 6% to 8%.[29,30] In addition, because 3 or more contributory factors are often present, the diagnostic workup should not be truncated after the identification of one reasonable cause of delirium.

Overall, delirium is a poor prognostic factor in cancer patients. Statistically significant decreases in median survival are reported in cancer patients with delirium compared with those without delirium, especially if the acute confusion is attributable to structural brain lesions or multiple toxic or metabolic abnormalities.[22,34–36]

Nonconvulsive Status Epilepticus

NCSE has been reported to be the underlying cause of altered mental status in up to 6% of cancer patients.[29,30] A high index of suspicion is required for the diagnosis of NCSE, in part due to its variable and nonspecific presentation, its lack of associated motor activity, and the absence of a prior history of epilepsy or seizures in most patients at presentation. NCSE is classically defined as a state of continuous or intermittent seizure activity without return to baseline lasting at least 30 minutes. More recently, the Epilepsy Research Foundation defined NCSE as a range of conditions in which electrographic seizure activity is prolonged, resulting in nonconvulsive clinical symptoms.[37]

The one consistent clinical symptom of NCSE is fluctuating altered mental status; however, even then, symptoms can encompass a spectrum ranging from psychomotor retardation to mild confusion to depressed consciousness. Motor manifestations are often limited to focal myoclonic jerks involving the face, eyelids, or extremities, however brief tonic or clonic movements of one or multiple extremities may also occur. Additional possible manifestations include head deviation, automatisms, and eye movement abnormalities including hippus, nystagmoid eye movements, repeated blinking, and persistent eye deviation. In one prospective study, the combination of a remote risk factor for seizures (previous stroke, neurosurgical procedure, brain tumor, or history of meningitis) and ocular movement abnormalities on neurologic examination had 100% sensitivity for NCSE, but low specificity.[38]

In some cases, imaging findings may support the diagnosis of NCSE. Characteristic cortical ribbon hyperintensity on long repetition time (TR)-weighted magnetic resonance sequences or diffusion weighted imaging sequences, with or without leptomeningeal enhancement was reported in 4 of 8 patients with NCSE in one series.[39] Imaging findings did not respect vascular territories, lacked mass effect, and either resolved or improved on follow-up imaging studies.[39]

Emergent electroencephalography (EEG) is recommended for patients with suspected NCSE. If an emergent EEG is not possible, an empirical trial of intravenous lorazepam should be considered given the tolerable risk of lorazepam compared with the benefit of potential prevention of secondary cerebral damage.

SEIZURES

New onset seizures herald the diagnosis of central nervous system brain tumors in 20% to 40% of patients, and account for 10% to 15% of adult-onset seizures.[40,41] Furthermore, seizures occur at some point in the clinical course in 40% to 60% of patients with gliomas, in 30% to 40% of patients with brain metastases, and in approximately 13% of all cancer patients.[3,40,42] Seizure risk varies depending on the tumor type and location, patient age, and tumor treatment.[42] Slow-growing tumors that involve or abut the cerebral cortex are associated with a higher incidence of seizures.[43]

In many cases, a clinical diagnosis of seizure is established after the patient history and examination is performed. However, disorders such as syncope, migraine, medication effects, and nonepileptic spells, may be confused with seizures. In addition, the diagnosis of NCSE is often overlooked in the ED. Head computed tomography (CT) and routine EEG should be considered as part of the neurodiagnostic evaluation of adult patients with unprovoked first seizure in the emergency department.[44,45] Brain imaging results in an acute management change in approximately 10% to 15% of these patients and EEG demonstrates significant abnormalities in approximately one third of patients, and provides risk assessment for seizure recurrence.[44,45]

Seizures associated with brain tumors and other structural lesions are most often simple partial or complex partial seizures. Secondarily generalized seizures may occur, but the focal onset of these seizures often goes unnoticed by the patient or witnesses. Postictal deficits (Todd's paralysis) are more common in patients with structural brain lesions and may be prolonged.[46] Whereas convulsive status epilepticus is rare in patients with brain tumors, it is fatal in 6% to 35%.[47] In contrast to structural seizures in brain tumor patients, seizures related to metabolic abnormalities are typically generalized seizures. Standard of care diagnostic evaluation and seizure management is appropriate in the brain tumor patient with the following specific considerations.

Many physicians endorse the prophylactic use of anticonvulsant medications in brain tumor patients who have never had a seizure, citing the high frequency of seizures in this patient population and the low risk of seizure medications. However, the emergency medicine physician must appreciate the lack of evidence that prophylactic anticonvulsant medications will prevent seizures in these patients, and that seizure medications are not without potential side effects and drug interactions. Phenytoin, a commonly prescribed anticonvulsant medication, causes a morbilliform rash in approximately 20% of brain tumor patients. Stevens-Johnson syndrome is rare, but is seen more often with the combination of radiation therapy, steroid taper, and phenytoin.[48] Even minor side effects of antiepileptic drug can negatively impact quality of life of patients already undergoing aggressive antitumor therapy. In addition, enzyme-inducing anticonvulsant medications may interact with chemotherapy and other drugs. For this reason, the use of nonenzyme-inducing anticonvulsant medications is preferable. Practice parameters issued by the American Academy of Neurology (AAN) currently recommend withholding prophylactic anticonvulsants in brain tumor patients who have never had a seizure.[42]

A related issue is the provision of prophylactic anticonvulsant medications in the setting of neurosurgical procedures. Traditionally, neurosurgeons prescribe prophylactic anticonvulsant medications before and for 6 to 12 weeks after neurosurgical procedures. The AAN practice guidelines recommend the tapering and discontinuance of anticonvulsant medications after the first postoperative week in brain tumor patients without known seizures.[42]

The etiology of provoked seizures in cancer patients is similar to that of the general population. However, some causes are particularly linked to cancer therapies. One such example is reversible posterior leukoencephalopathy syndrome (RPLS), also known as posterior reversible encephalopathy syndrome. RPLS in cancer patients is associated with numerous chemotherapeutic agents, especially cisplatin. RPLS has also been reported following the administration of 5-fluorouracil, bleomycin, vinblastine, vincristine, etoposide, paclitaxel, ifosfamide, cyclophosphamide, doxorubicin, cytarabine, methotrexate, oxaliplatin, and bevacizumab.[49–51]

The classic presentation of RPLS is the development of a subacute syndrome of headache, altered consciousness, generalized seizures, and visual disturbances, occurring in conjunction with posterior cerebral white matter vasogenic edema on CT/MRI.[52] Typically the syndrome manifests over several days, but a more acute presentation may occur. Altered consciousness may vary from excessive drowsiness to coma, seizures may be focal or generalized, and visual disturbances range from blurred vision to cortical blindness. Additional neurologic symptoms such as paresis may also be present. Moderate to severe hypertension occurs in approximately 75% of patients. Hypertension typically develops at the same time as neurologic symptoms, but occasionally it may precede the clinical manifestations of RPLS.[53,54]

Radiographically, MRI typically demonstrates symmetric hemispheric edema in the parietal and occipital lobes involving cortical and subcortical white matter, approximating the border zone vascular territory.[54] Although involvement of the parietal and occipital lobes occurs most often, similar radiographic abnormalities can be located in the frontal lobes, the inferior temporal-occipital junction, and the cerebellum. Focal areas of restricted diffusion are seen in less than one fourth of patients. Approximately 15% of patients have radiographic evidence of hemorrhage in the form of focal hematoma, or isolated sulcal or subarachnoid blood.[54]

ACUTE STROKE

Ischemic, hemorrhagic, and thrombotic cerebrovascular disease occurs in approximately 15% of cancer patients, but only one half of cancer patients experience symptoms referable to their lesions.[55] Most cerebrovascular disease associated with hematologic cancer is hemorrhagic, whereas in solid tumors there is an even division between infarction and hemorrhage.[55]

Cerebral infarction occurs infrequently in hematologic malignancies, and is generally hemorrhagic. Leukemic patients may develop septic emboli, infarction related to disseminated intravascular coagulation, or venous infarctions related to cerebral venous thrombosis. Most cerebral infarction in patients with lymphoma is attributable to disseminated intravascular coagulation or nonbacterial thrombotic endocarditis (NBTE).

Most strokes in patients with solid tumors are embolic and tend to occur late in the patient's clinical course. Rarely, stroke can be the presenting symptom of occult malignancy.[56–58] NBTE is frequently cited as the most common cause of stroke in cancer patients, and some propose that cancer-specific factors such as tumor type and associated coagulation disorders are more determinant of stroke risk in cancer patients than the classic atherosclerotic stroke risk factors.[55,59] However, supporting data are inconsistent. Whereas some reports attribute a disproportionately small number of strokes in cancer patients, less than 20%, to atherosclerotic disease, other studies report no significant difference in atherosclerotic stroke incidence between cancer stroke patients and noncancer stroke patients.[55,59–62] Overall, the ED physician must consider typical ischemic stroke mechanisms as well as disease-specific stroke risk factors in the cancer patient. The more common cancer-related stroke mechanisms are discussed in the following subsections.

Nonbacterial Thrombotic Endocarditis

NBTE is characterized by the presence of cardiac valve vegetation formed by fibrin and platelet aggregates, occurring in the absence of infection or inflammation. Involvement of left-sided heart valves (aortic more often than mitral) is more common than right-sided heart valves.[63] The vegetation is typically small, irregular, and easily friable with a strong propensity to embolize.[64] Not surprisingly, the most common presenting symptom, occurring in approximately 50% of patients, is recurrent systemic emboli to cerebral, coronary, renal, and mesenteric bed circulations or the extremities, respectively producing acute stroke, myocardial infarction, hematuria, abdominal pain, or cold, cyanotic, or pulseless limbs.[63,64] Symptomatic valvular dysfunction is uncommon.

NBTE is most commonly associated with widely disseminated mucin-producing adenocarcinomas of the lung or gastrointestinal tract and lymphoma.[64,65] Approximately 70% of patients have coexistent disseminated intravascular coagulation.[66] Autopsy data suggest that NBTE often goes undiagnosed in the clinical setting, reflecting the difficulty in establishing a definitive diagnosis.[59] The diagnostic gold standard is the demonstration of valvular vegetation on transesophageal echocardiogram in the absence of positive blood cultures. However, due to the nature of the vegetation and its propensity to embolize, transesophageal echocardiogram may not detect the remaining small, fragmented vegetation. Additional clues may be of diagnostic importance in the cancer patient. Whereas cardiac murmurs are uncommon in NBTE, their presence in a cancer patient should raise a diagnostic suspicion of NBTE. Likewise, abnormal coagulation studies, including prothrombin time, partial thromboplastin time, fibrinogen, thrombin time, D-dimer, and cross-linked fibrin degradation products are suggestive of NBTE in the appropriate clinical setting. The distribution of strokes on brain MRI may be helpful in differentiating NBTE from septic emboli. One small study found that strokes due to NBTE involved multiple, widespread, small and large arteries, as opposed to a single lesion, multiple lesions within a single arterial territory, or multiple punctate disseminated lesions—all patterns more suggestive of septic emboli.[67] If feasible, the treatment of NBTE is typically life-long anticoagulation with intravenous or subcutaneous heparin.[68] Warfarin often fails to control the coagulopathy and is associated with recurrent thromboembolic events.[68] There are insufficient data for comment on the efficacy of the newer anticoagulant agents such as fondaparinux.

Therapy-Induced Stroke

Cerebrovascular disease may be provoked by cancer therapy. In fact, cancer treatment accounts for most strokes in patients with a primary brain tumor. Approximately 20% to 60% of strokes in this patient population are the result of intraoperative vascular injury and occur adjacent to the resection bed.[62,69] In addition, brain irradiation commonly causes accelerated atherosclerosis and small vessel arteriopathy within the radiated field, which may cause stroke or transient ischemic attacks in medium to large vessels typically occurring 6 months to 5 years following radiation treatment.[62,70,71] Conventional atherosclerotic stroke management is appropriate in these patients.

Ischemic stroke occurs in less than 1% of cancer patients receiving chemotherapy, primarily L-asparaginase, cisplatin, 5-fluorouracil, and methotrexate.[72–75] Mechanisms include thrombosis, vasospasm, thrombocytopenia, and decreased renewal capacity of endothelial cells. Despite the wide range of proposed causes, the vascular events related to chemotherapy almost always occur within days to 1 month of therapy.

Tumor Emboli

Solid tumors rarely produce stroke as the result of tumor emboli to cerebral arteries, compression or invasion of a cerebral artery, or compression of cerebral sinuses causing venous infarction.[76,77] The most common sources of tumor emboli are atrial myxomas and other cardiac tumors, as well as lung cancer. Lung tumor emboli most often occur within 48 hours of surgical manipulation of lung tissue, but may also result from tumor invasion of the pulmonary veins or left atrium of the heart.[76] Signs and symptoms of emboli to multiple body organs or the extremities are frequently seen. Stroke from lung tumor emboli should be suspected in any patient with primary or metastatic lung cancer who develops stroke in the immediate postoperative period or has evidence of multi-organ infarction. Treatment must address tumor growth at the embolic infarction site and the primary tumor.

Septic Emboli

Leukemia patients are particularly susceptible to septic infarction from fungal or bacterial sepsis and infectious vasculitis. Agranulocytosis during and after therapy predisposes these patients to fungal infection, in particular *Aspergillus* or *Candida* sp.[78] *Aspergillus* pulmonary infection facilitates hematogenous dissemination of these microorganisms, and their large hyphae may become trapped with the lumen of medium- to large-sized vessels, causing cerebral infarction and focal neurologic deficits.[79] Infarctions are often multiple, may be hemorrhagic, and may evolve into cerebral abscess. Chest roentgenograms or CT scans often indicate infection, and patients may be febrile. Blood and sputum cultures are typically negative. Transbronchial biopsy or brain biopsy is often necessary to establish the diagnosis. Antifungal therapy is often ineffective and patients generally succumb to progressive infection.

Hemorrhagic Cerebral Metastases

Hemorrhage into cerebral metastases in patients with melanoma, germ cell, and non-small-cell lung carcinoma primaries account for most hemorrhagic cerebrovascular disease in patients with solid tumors.[55] Thrombocytopenia-related intracranial hemorrhage occurs less commonly. Hemorrhage into a solid tumor causes acute strokelike symptoms in two thirds of patients and subacute focal neurologic symptoms suggestive of an enlarging mass lesion in one third of patients. In contrast to primary intracerebral hemorrhage, corticosteroids are beneficial in intratumoral hemorrhage.[80] Surgical evacuation of the clot may be indicated to reduce increased intracranial pressure. Additional treatment addresses the underlying metastatic disease.

Pituitary Apoplexy

Pituitary apoplexy is an acute, potentially life-threatening clinical syndrome caused by the acute expansion of a hypophyseal adenoma as a result of hemorrhage or infarction. It occurs in 0.6% to 17% of patients with pituitary adenoma, in particular chromophobic and eosinophilic adenomas.[81,82] However, intralesional hemorrhage or infarct may be asymptomatic and only evident on radiographic studies or at microscopic examination. Apoplexy is rarely the presenting symptom of a pituitary adenoma.[81,83] Predisposing factors include conditions that either reduce or acutely increase blood flow in the pituitary gland, hormonal stimulation of the pituitary gland, or anticoagulated states.[84]

Clinically, acute expansion of the pituitary gland and compression of perisellar structures may cause severe headaches, nausea, vomiting, visual disturbances, ophthalmoplegia, and decreased level of consciousness. Long-standing pituitary gland compression may result in hypopituitarism. Prompt surgical decompression is indicated in acutely symptomatic cases.[83] Medical management may be considered in appropriate tumor subtypes with more indolent clinical presentations.

LEPTOMENINGEAL METASTASES

Leptomeningeal metastases (LM) occurs in up to 8% of all cancer patients, and in 5% to 20% of cancer patients with widely metastatic disease.[85,86] Primary brain tumors, such as primary lymphomas, medulloblastomas, and germ cell tumors of the central nervous system, may have LM at initial diagnosis.[87] Otherwise, LM rarely occurs in patients without evidence of widespread systemic disease.[88,89] Any systemic cancer can spread to the leptomeninges; however, LM is most commonly associated with leukemia, non-Hodgkin lymphoma, breast carcinoma, non-small-cell lung cancer, and melanoma.[90–92]

The clinical hallmark of LM is the presence of symptoms and signs referable to multiple sites within the central nervous system, cranial nerves, and spinal roots. Not surprisingly, the presentation of LM is highly variable and diagnosis requires a high index of suspicion. Virtually any nervous system abnormality may occur; however, some symptoms are seen more consistently. Approximately 60% of patients with LM report weakness and paresthesia of the lower extremities indicating lumbosacral nerve root involvement, and more than 70% will have corresponding spinal signs of asymmetric weakness, sensory loss, and depressed reflexes. One half of patients manifest nonspecific cerebral symptoms including headache, nausea and vomiting, and cognitive changes. Meningismus and nuchal rigidity are present in only 15% of patients. One third of patients have cranial nerve dysfunction. In decreasing frequency, patients have symptoms and signs of oculomotor, facial, auditory, optic, trigeminal, and hypoglossal nerve dysfunction.[90–92] Papilledema may occur in the setting of communicating hydrocephalus. Uncommon manifestations of LM include diabetes insipidus, central hypoventilation, cerebral infarction, NCSE, and psychiatric symptoms.[93]

A definitive diagnosis of LM requires identification of malignant cells in the cerebrospinal fluid (CSF). Two or 3 samplings of CSF may be required before malignant cells are detected; the diagnostic yield of CSF samples obtained in the ED can be optimized through the collection of at least 10 mL of CSF for cytologic examination, and the prompt delivery of the specimen to the laboratory. Characteristic CSF abnormalities in LM include an elevated opening pressure in more than 50% of patients, mononuclear pleocytosis in more than 70% of patients, elevated protein in approximately 80% of patients, and decreased glucose in 25% to 30% of patients. The range of CSF protein elevation in LM is wide with a median total protein concentration of 1 g/L.[94]

In some cases, a presumptive diagnosis of LM is made on the basis of appropriate clinical symptoms and signs and neuroimaging findings consistent with LM in known cancer patients. MRI diagnosis of LM has up to 65% sensitivity and 77% specificity.[93] MR findings in LM may be normal or may demonstrate communicating hydrocephalus, effacement of the sulci and cisterns, linear or nodular subependymal, leptomeningeal, nerve root, or dural enhancement, and diffuse thickening of spinal nerve roots.[95] Diffuse leptomeningeal enhancement can also occur with cerebral hypotension following lumbar puncture, and may be misinterpreted as radiographic evidence of LM.[96] For this reason, if feasible, MRI should be obtained before lumbar puncture.

The overall prognosis of LM is poor; however, the cause of death in these patients is most often widespread uncontrolled systemic disease, not LM. As a consequence, the primary expectation of treatment is improved quality of life and prolonged time to neurologic progression.[97] The treatment of LM must address the entire neuroaxis and relies on a combination of radiation, chemotherapy, and supportive care. Radiation provides the most effective symptom relief and therapy for bulky tumor deposits. However, irradiation of the entire neuroaxis is generally too toxic in heavily pretreated patients. Chemotherapy provided by either intrathecal (IT) injection or systemic routes on occasion addresses LM disease throughout the entire neuroaxis.[97–99] However, impairment of CSF flow, which occurs in up to 70% of patients with LM, can impede uniform IT chemotherapy distribution and is a significant factor in drug failure.[100] Therefore, a combined approach is typically used consisting of chemotherapy and focal irradiation targeting regions of bulky disease, symptomatic levels of the neuro-axis, and regions of subarachnoid CSF block.[101]

Acute therapy complications frequently prompt ED evaluation. The most common complication, aseptic meningitis, clinically mimics bacterial meningitis. Similar to bacterial meningitis, CSF analysis shows pleocytosis and elevated protein. However, aseptic meningitis occurs within hours to 1 day following IT drug administration, much earlier than one would see iatrogenic bacterial meningitis. Symptoms generally resolve within a few days and treatment is symptomatic with antipyretics, antiemetics, and steroids. Aseptic meningitis may occur following the first IT drug dose or after any number of cycles. The syndrome often does not recur and further IT treatment may be provided.

Acute encephalopathy characterized by seizures, altered mental status, and leth-argy, may occur within 24 to 48 hours of IT MTX or AraC. The treatment is symptomatic and symptoms generally resolve completely. In addition, concurrent IT chemotherapy and spinal irradiation may cause a transverse myelopathy. Back or leg pain, para-plegia, sensory loss, and bowel/bladder dysfunction typically develop within 48 hours of IT chemotherapy, but may occur within 30 minutes or up to 2 weeks following treat-ment. CSF is found to have elevated protein levels and MRI shows expansion of the spinal cord and hyperintensity on T2-weighted sequences. The prognosis for recovery is poor with persistent paraparesis in approximately 60% of those affected.

PARANEOPLASTIC NEUROLOGIC SYNDROMES

Paraneoplastic neurologic syndromes (PNS) are a collective group of disorders occur-ring in patients with cancer as a remote effect of the malignancy. These syndromes cannot be attributed directly to the tumor or its metastases, to cancer therapies, or to cancer-associated infection, vascular or coagulation disorders, nutritional deficits, or metabolic abnormalities (**Table 2**). PNS develop in 3% to 5% of patients with small-cell lung cancer, in 15% to 20% with thymomas, and in 3% to 10% with B cell or plasma cell neoplasms.[102] They occur in less than 1% of other tumor types.[102] Overall, PNS are diagnosed in less than 0.01% of cancer patients.[103] However, despite their rarity, paraneoplastic disorders have a significant impact on oncology patients not only because they antedate the diagnosis of cancer in up to 80% of affected individ-uals but also because they frequently cause significant disability due to early onset and irreversible destruction of neural tissues.[104] Prompt recognition of PNS by the emergency medicine physician will help facilitate an accurate diagnosis, allowing treatment of the underlying tumor at an early stage, and potentially mitigating neuro-logic disability.

Critical to the diagnosis of PNS is the recognition of a specific group of neurologic syndromes, referred to as classic PNS, that are highly suggestive, but not diagnostic, of a paraneoplastic origin. These classic PNS include Lambert-Eaton myasthenic syndrome, subacute cerebellar degeneration, limbic encephalitis, sensory neuronop-athy, opsoclonus-myoclonus, dermatomyositis, stiff-person syndrome, retinopathy, encephalomyelitis, and chronic gastrointestinal pseudo-obstruction. However, it is important for the emergency medicine physician to recognize that most patients with these syndromes do not harbor an underlying malignancy. Approximately 50% of patients with Lambert-Eaton myasthenic syndrome or subacute cerebellar degen-eration have an underlying tumor, whereas the incidence of malignancy in the remain-ing classic PNS is less than 20%.[104] Several factors implicate paraneoplastic origin.

Table 2
Classic paraneoplastic neurologic syndromes

Classic PNS	Onset	Primary Clinical Symptoms and Signs
Limbic encephalitis	Subacute over weeks to months	o Short term memory loss that may progress to dementia o Personality changes o Anxiety, depression. agitation o Confusion o Olfactory and gustatory hallucinations o Partial or generalized seizures o Sleep disturbances
Subacute cerebellar degeneration	Subacute over weeks to months	o Initially patients note gait instability, then rapid evolution to truncal and limb ataxia o Dysarthria and dysphagia o Diplopia and nystagmus
Opsoclonus–myoclonus	Fairly acute over days to weeks	o Opsoclonus (almost continuous involuntary, arrhythmic, multidirectional chaotic rapid eye movements, that persist during eye closure and sleep) o Myoclonic jerks of limbs and trunk o Mild encephalopathy
Cancer-associated retinopathy (CAR)	Subacute over weeks to months	o Painless vision loss progressing to blindness over 6 to 18 months o Photopsias (flickering lights) o Peripheral and ring scotomatas
Melanoma-associated retinopathy(MAR)	Acute over days	o Shimmering or flickering light phenomena o Night blindness o Midperipheral visual field loss
Stiff-person syndrome	Insidious	o Rigidity of axial and proximal limb muscles with cocontraction of agonist and antagonist muscles o Intermittent painful spasms precipitated by sensory stimuli o Symptoms are absent during sleep and anesthesia

Subacute sensory neuronopathy	Subacute	○ Asymmetric pain and paresthesias involving the arms more than the legs ○ Pain is later replaced by numbness, limb ataxia, and pseudoathetotic movements of the hands ○ Facial numbness, sensorineural deafness, and sensory abnormalities of the trunk may also occur ○ Absent deep tendon reflexes and involvement of all sensory modalities especially joint position and vibratory senses
Chronic gastrointestinal pseudo-obstruction	Subacute	○ Severe constipation ○ Weight loss ○ Abdominal distension ○ Dysphagia ○ Nausea and vomiting
Lambert-Eaton myasthenic syndrome	Subacute	○ Proximal muscle weakness, legs more than arms. Symptoms are out of proportion to weakness. Strength may initially improve after exercise then decrease with sustained activity. Deep tendon reflexes are reduced or absent, but may transiently improve after exercise. ○ Mild autonomic dysfunction ○ Mild ptosis/ophthalmoplegia
Dermatomyositis	Slowly progressive over months	○ Symmetric proximal muscle weakness ○ Associated cutaneous manifestations include a heliotrope rash involving the peri-orbital skin, erythematous scaly plaques on dorsal hands, periungual telangiectasia, Gottron's papules, and a photosensitive poikilodermatous eruption

The presence of risk factors for malignancy such as smoking or family history, or symptoms associated with malignancy such as unexplained weight loss or night sweats, warrants consideration of a paraneoplastic origin. The presentation and disease course of PNS is often dramatic compared with the corresponding non–tumor-related syndromes. PNS typically have a subacute symptom onset with a rapidly progressive clinical course and early onset of severe disability.[105] In addition, syndromic overlap is frequently seen in PNS, but uncommon in disorders unrelated to cancer.

By definition, a paraneoplastic neurologic disorder requires the presence of an underlying malignancy, generally within 5 years of its diagnosis. Most patients do not have an established cancer diagnosis at presentation; however, the underlying cancer is discovered in 70% to 80% of patients at the initial cancer screening or within 4 to 6 months.[102] The risk of developing cancer significantly decreases after 2 years and becomes remote after 5 years. CT of the chest, abdomen, and pelvis or fluorodeoxyglucose positron emission tomography are the most commonly used screening tests for malignancy in cases of suspected PNS.

In many cases, patients with PNS may either present with a nonclassic neurologic syndrome or have no identifiable tumor. In these scenarios, the identification of a well-characterized paraneoplastic antibody facilitates the definite diagnosis of PNS. Although numerous paraneoplastic or onconeural antibodies are currently under investigation for a purported relationship with PNS, only a few have been well characterized, including anti-Hu (antinuclear neuronal antibody type 1 or ANNA-1), anti-Yo (Purkinje cell antibody type 1 or PCA-1), anti-Ri (ANNA-2), anti-CV2/CRMP5, anti-Ma proteins, and anti-amphyphysin. However, up to 50% of patients with an established PNS diagnosis do not have detectable paraneoplastic antibodies.[105] Additional corroborating clinical evidence is required to establish a diagnosis of possible PNS in those patients with clinically suspected PNS that does not meet the diagnostic criteria.

Aside from onconeural antibodies, the diagnostic workup for paraneoplastic disorders yields fairly nonspecific findings of central nervous system inflammation, and, most importantly, serves to exclude alternative disorders. CSF evaluation may show mild pleocytosis, elevated protein, and oligoclonal bands. Histopathologic tissue examination demonstrates a nonspecific T cell infiltration.[102] Brain MRI is typically normal. However, hyperintensity on long TR sequences involving the mesial temporal lobes can be seen in limbic encephalitis. More widespread abnormalities, with additional involvement of the brain stem, may be seen in patients with encephalomyelitis. Cerebellar atrophy is a late finding in subacute cerebellar degeneration.

To date, there are no evidence-based recommendations for treatment of PNS. Successful treatment of the underlying malignancy is by far the most effective treatment strategy for the stabilization of neurologic deficits from PNS. Immune therapy is often beneficial for PNS affecting the peripheral nervous system, neuromuscular junction, and muscle, and may consist of steroids, intravenous immunoglobulin, or plasma exchange. Central nervous system paraneoplastic disorders are more refractory to treatment, although there are anecdotal reports of response to steroids or intravenous immunoglobulin, as well as spontaneous remission. Symptomatic treatment of seizures, psychiatric manifestations, movement disorders, and so forth is indicated.

REFERENCES

1. Swenson KK, Rose MA, Ritz L, et al. Recognition and evaluation of oncology-related symptoms in the emergency department. Ann Emerg Med 1995;26: 12–7.

2. Gilbert MR, Grossman SA. Incidence and nature of neurologic problems in patients with solid tumors. Am J Med 1986;81:951–4.
3. Clouston PD, DeAngelis LM, Posner JB. The spectrum of neurological disease in patients with systemic cancer. Ann Neurol 1992;31:268–73.
4. Black P, Wen P. Clinical, imaging and laboratory diagnosis of brain tumors. In: Kaye AH, Laws E Jr, editors. Brain tumors. New York: Churchill Livingstone; 1995. p. 191–214.
5. Matsuda M, Yoneda S, Handa H, et al. Cerebral hemodynamic changes during plateau waves in brain-tumor patients. J Neurosurg 1979;50:483–8.
6. Gassel MM. False localizing signs. A review of the concept and analysis of the occurrence in 250 cases of intracranial meningioma. Arch Neurol 1961;4: 526–54.
7. Sarin R, Murthy V. Medical decompressive therapy for primary and metastatic intracranial tumours. Lancet Neurol 2003;2:357–65.
8. Weissman DE. Glucocorticoid treatment for brain metastases and epidural spinal cord compression: a review. J Clin Oncol 1988;6:543–51.
9. Ruderman NB, Hall TC. Use of glucocorticoids in the palliative treatment of metastatic brain tumors. Cancer 1965;18:298–306.
10. Alberti E, Hartmann A, Schutz HJ, et al. The effect of large doses of dexamethasone on the cerebrospinal fluid pressure in patients with supratentorial tumors. J Neurol 1978;217:173–81.
11. Lieberman A, LeBrun Y, Glass P, et al. Use of high dose corticosteroids in patients with inoperable brain tumours. J Neurol Neurosurg Psychiatr 1977;40: 678–82.
12. Renaudin J, Fewer D, Wilson CB, et al. Dose dependency of decadron in patients with partially excised brain tumors. J Neurosurg 1973;39:302–5.
13. Ropper AH, Gress DR, Diringer MN, et al. Management of intracranial pressure and mass effect. In: Ropper AH, editor. Neurological and neurosurgical intensive care. 4th edition. Philadelphia: Lippincott Williams & Wilkins; 2003. p. 26–51.
14. The Brain Trauma Foundation, The American Association of Neurological Surgeons, The Joint Section on Neurotrauma and Critical Care. Use of mannitol. J Neurotrauma 2000;17:521–5.
15. Koenig MA, Bryan M, Lewin JL 3rd, et al. Reversal of transtentorial herniation with hypertonic saline. Neurology 2008;70:1023–9.
16. Ravussin P, Abou-Madi M, Archer D, et al. Changes in CSF pressure after mannitol in patients with and without elevated CSF pressure. J Neurosurg 1988;69:869–76.
17. Pollay M, Fullenwider C, Roberts PA, et al. Effect of mannitol and furosemide on blood-brain osmotic gradient and intracranial pressure. J Neurosurg 1983;59: 945–50.
18. Vialet R, Albanese J, Thomachot L, et al. Isovolume hypertonic solutes (sodium chloride or mannitol) in the treatment of refractory posttraumatic intracranial hypertension: 2 mL/kg 7.5% saline is more effective than 2 mL/kg 20% mannitol. Crit Care Med 2003;31:1683–7.
19. Qureshi AI, Suarez JI. Use of hypertonic saline solutions in treatment of cerebral edema and intracranial hypertension. Crit Care Med 2000;28:3301–13.
20. Suarez JI, Qureshi AI, Bhardwaj A, et al. Treatment of refractory intracranial hypertension with 23.4% saline. Crit Care Med 1998;26:1118–22.
21. Alkire MT, Haier RJ, Barker SJ, et al. Cerebral metabolism during propofol anesthesia in humans studied with positron emission tomography. Anesthesiology 1995;82:393–403 [discussion: 27A].

22. Lawlor PG, Gagnon B, Mancini IL, et al. Occurrence, causes, and outcome of delirium in patients with advanced cancer: a prospective study. Arch Intern Med 2000;160:786–94.
23. Doriath V, Paesmans M, Catteau G, et al. Acute confusion in patients with systemic cancer. J Neurooncol 2007;83:285–9.
24. Tuma R, DeAngelis LM. Altered mental status in patients with cancer. Arch Neurol 2000;57:1727–31.
25. Weinrich S, Sarna L. Delirium in the older person with cancer. Cancer 1994;74: 2079–91.
26. Marcantonio ER, Goldman L, Mangione CM, et al. A clinical prediction rule for delirium after elective noncardiac surgery. JAMA 1994;271:134–9.
27. Francis J, Martin D, Kapoor WN. A prospective study of delirium in hospitalized elderly. JAMA 1990;263:1097–101.
28. Schor JD, Levkoff SE, Lipsitz LA, et al. Risk factors for delirium in hospitalized elderly. JAMA 1992;267:827–31.
29. Cocito L, Audenino D, Primavera A. Altered mental state and nonconvulsive status epilepticus in patients with cancer. Arch Neurol 2001;58:1310.
30. Towne AR, Waterhouse EJ, Boggs JG, et al. Prevalence of nonconvulsive status epilepticus in comatose patients. Neurology 2000;54:340–5.
31. Maddocks I, Somogyi A, Abbott F, et al. Attenuation of morphine-induced delirium in palliative care by substitution with infusion of oxycodone. J Pain Symptom Manage 1996;12:182–9.
32. de Stoutz ND, Bruera E, Suarez-Almazor M. Opioid rotation for toxicity reduction in terminal cancer patients. J Pain Symptom Manage 1995;10:378–84.
33. Inouye SK, Charpentier PA. Precipitating factors for delirium in hospitalized elderly persons. Predictive model and interrelationship with baseline vulnerability. JAMA 1996;275:852–7.
34. Massie MJ, Holland J, Glass E. Delirium in terminally ill cancer patients. Am J Psychiatry 1983;140:1048–50.
35. Fang CK, Chen HW, Liu SI, et al. Prevalence, detection and treatment of delirium in terminal cancer inpatients: a prospective survey. Jpn J Clin Oncol 2008;38: 56–63.
36. Caraceni A, Nanni O, Maltoni M, et al. Impact of delirium on the short term prognosis of advanced cancer patients. Italian Multicenter Study Group on Palliative Care. Cancer 2000;89:1145–9.
37. Walker M, Cross H, Smith S, et al. Nonconvulsive status epilepticus: Epilepsy Research Foundation workshop reports. Epileptic Disord 2005;7:253–96.
38. Husain AM, Horn GJ, Jacobson MP. Non-convulsive status epilepticus: usefulness of clinical features in selecting patients for urgent EEG. J Neurol Neurosurg Psychiatr 2003;74:189–91.
39. Hormigo A, Liberato B, Lis E, et al. Nonconvulsive status epilepticus in patients with cancer: imaging abnormalities. Arch Neurol 2004;61:362–5.
40. Cohen N, Strauss G, Lew R, et al. Should prophylactic anticonvulsants be administered to patients with newly-diagnosed cerebral metastases? A retrospective analysis. J Clin Oncol 1988;6:1621–4.
41. van Breemen MS, Wilms EB, Vecht CJ. Epilepsy in patients with brain tumours: epidemiology, mechanisms, and management. Lancet Neurol 2007;6:421–30.
42. Glantz MJ, Cole BF, Forsyth PA, et al. Practice parameter: anticonvulsant prophylaxis in patients with newly diagnosed brain tumors. Report of the Quality Standards Subcommittee of the American Academy of Neurology. Neurology 2000;54:1886–93.

43. Hughes JR, Zak SM. EEG and clinical changes in patients with chronic seizures associated with slowly growing brain tumors. Arch Neurol 1987;44:540–3.
44. Harden CL, Huff JS, Schwartz TH, et al. Reassessment: Neuroimaging in the emergency patient presenting with seizure (an evidence-based review): report of the Therapeutics and Technology Assessment Subcommittee of the American Academy of Neurology. Neurology 2007;69:1772–80.
45. Krumholz A, Wiebe S, Gronseth G, et al. Practice parameter: evaluating an apparent unprovoked first seizure in adults (an evidence-based review): report of the Quality Standards Subcommittee of the American Academy of Neurology and the American Epilepsy Society. Neurology 2007;69:1996–2007.
46. Forsyth PA, Weaver S, Fulton D, et al. Prophylactic anticonvulsants in patients with brain tumour. Can J Neurol Sci 2003;30:106–12.
47. Engel J. Seizures and epilepsy. Philadelphia: F.A. Davis Co; 1989.
48. Delattre JY, Safai B, Posner JB. Erythema multiforme and Stevens-Johnson syndrome in patients receiving cranial irradiation and phenytoin. Neurology 1988;38:194–8.
49. Skelton MR, Goldberg RM, O'Neil BH. A case of oxaliplatin-related posterior reversible encephalopathy syndrome. Clin Colorectal Cancer 2007;6:386–8.
50. Ozcan C, Wong SJ, Hari P. Reversible posterior leukoencephalopathy syndrome and bevacizumab. N Engl J Med 2006;354:980–2 [discussion: 2].
51. Glusker P, Recht L, Lane B. Reversible posterior leukoencephalopathy syndrome and bevacizumab. N Engl J Med 2006;354:980–2 [discussion: 2].
52. Hinchey J, Chaves C, Appignani B, et al. A reversible posterior leukoencephalopathy syndrome. N Engl J Med 1996;334:494–500.
53. Stott VL, Hurrell MA, Anderson TJ. Reversible posterior leukoencephalopathy syndrome: a misnomer reviewed. Intern Med J 2005;35:83–90.
54. Bartynski WS. Posterior reversible encephalopathy syndrome, part 1: fundamental imaging and clinical features. AJNR Am J Neuroradiol 2008;29:1036–42.
55. Graus F, Rogers LR, Posner JB. Cerebrovascular complications in patients with cancer. Medicine (Baltimore) 1985;64:16–35.
56. Perez-Lazaro C, Santos S, Morales-Rull JL, et al. Letus como primera manifestación de una neoplasia pancreática oculta [Stroke as the first manifestation of a concealed pancreatic neoplasia]. Rev Neurol 2004;38:332–5.
57. Taccone FS, Jeangette SM, Blecic SA. First-ever stroke as initial presentation of systemic cancer. J Stroke Cerebrovasc Dis 2008;17:169–74.
58. Kwon HM, Kang BS, Yoon BW. Stroke as the first manifestation of concealed cancer. J Neurol Sci 2007;258:80–3.
59. Cestari DM, Weine DM, Panageas KS, et al. Stroke in patients with cancer: incidence and etiology. Neurology 2004;62:2025–30.
60. Chaturvedi S, Ansell J, Recht L. Should cerebral ischemic events in cancer patients be considered a manifestation of hypercoagulability? Stroke 1994;25:1215–8.
61. Zhang YY, Chan DK, Cordato D, et al. Stroke risk factor, pattern and outcome in patients with cancer. Acta Neurol Scand 2006;114:378–83.
62. Kreisl TN, Toothaker T, Karimi S, et al. Ischemic stroke in patients with primary brain tumors. Neurology 2008;70:2314–20.
63. el-Shami K, Griffiths E, Streiff M. Nonbacterial thrombotic endocarditis in cancer patients: pathogenesis, diagnosis, and treatment. Oncologist 2007;12:518–23.
64. Asopa S, Patel A, Khan OA, et al. Non-bacterial thrombotic endocarditis. Eur J Cardiothorac Surg 2007;32:696–701.

65. Edoute Y, Haim N, Rinkevich D, et al. Cardiac valvular vegetations in cancer patients: a prospective echocardiographic study of 200 patients. Am J Med 1997;102:252–8.

66. Bedikian A, Valdivieso M, Luna M, et al. Nonbacterial thrombotic endocarditis in cancer patients: comparison of characteristics of patients with and without concomitant disseminated intravascular coagulation. Med Pediatr Oncol 1978; 4:149–57.

67. Singhal AB, Topcuoglu MA, Buonanno FS. Acute ischemic stroke patterns in infective and nonbacterial thrombotic endocarditis: a diffusion-weighted magnetic resonance imaging study. Stroke 2002;33:1267–73.

68. Rogers LR, Cho ES, Kempin S, et al. Cerebral infarction from non-bacterial thrombotic endocarditis. Clinical and pathological study including the effects of anticoagulation. Am J Med 1987;83:746–56.

69. Smith JS, Cha S, Mayo MC, et al. Serial diffusion-weighted magnetic resonance imaging in cases of glioma: distinguishing tumor recurrence from postresection injury. J Neurosurg 2005;103:428–38.

70. Murros KE, Toole JF. The effect of radiation on carotid arteries. A review article. Arch Neurol 1989;46:449–55.

71. Bowers DC, Liu Y, Leisenring W, et al. Late-occurring stroke among long-term survivors of childhood leukemia and brain tumors: a report from the Childhood Cancer Survivor Study. J Clin Oncol 2006;24:5277–82.

72. Li SH, Chen WH, Tang Y, et al. Incidence of ischemic stroke post-chemotherapy: a retrospective review of 10,963 patients. Clin Neurol Neurosurg 2006;108:150–6.

73. Czaykowski PM, Moore MJ, Tannock IF. High risk of vascular events in patients with urothelial transitional cell carcinoma treated with cisplatin based chemotherapy. J Urol 1998;160:2021–4.

74. Saynak M, Cosar-Alas R, Yurut-Caloglu V, et al. Chemotherapy and cerebrovascular disease. J BUON 2008;13:31–6.

75. Wall JG, Weiss RB, Norton L, et al. Arterial thrombosis associated with adjuvant chemotherapy for breast carcinoma: a Cancer and Leukemia Group B Study. Am J Med 1989;87:501–4.

76. Lefkovitz NW, Roessmann U, Kori SH. Major cerebral infarction from tumor embolus. Stroke 1986;17:555–7.

77. Klein P, Haley EC, Wooten GF, et al. Focal cerebral infarctions associated with perivascular tumor infiltrates in carcinomatous leptomeningeal metastases. Arch Neurol 1989;46:1149–52.

78. Kawanami T, Kurita K, Yamakawa M, et al. Cerebrovascular disease in acute leukemia: a clinicopathological study of 14 patients. Intern Med 2002;41:1130–4.

79. Scaravilli FC, Cook GC. Parasitis and fungal infections. In: Graham DI, Lantos D, editors. 6th edition, Greenfield's neuropathology, vol. 2. London: Arnold; 1997. p. 543–8.

80. Poungvarin N, Bhoopat W, Viriyavejakul A, et al. Effects of dexamethasone in primary supratentorial intracerebral hemorrhage. N Engl J Med 1987;316: 1229–33.

81. Cardoso ER, Peterson EW. Pituitary apoplexy: a review. Neurosurgery 1984;14: 363–73.

82. Symon L, Mohanty S. Haemorrhage in pituitary tumours. Acta Neurochir (Wien) 1982;65:41–9.

83. Ebersold MJ, Laws ER Jr, Scheithauer BW, et al. Pituitary apoplexy treated by transsphenoidal surgery. A clinicopathological and immunocytochemical study. J Neurosurg 1983;58:315–20.

84. Biousse V, Newman NJ, Oyesiku NM. Precipitating factors in pituitary apoplexy. J Neurol Neurosurg Psychiatr 2001;71:542–5.

85. Chamberlain MC, Kormanik PA, Barba D. Complications associated with intraventricular chemotherapy in patients with leptomeningeal metastases. J Neurosurg 1997;87:694–9.

86. Olson ME, Chernik NL, Posner JB. Infiltration of the leptomeninges by systemic cancer. A clinical and pathologic study. Arch Neurol 1974;30:122–37.

87. Engelhard HH, Corsten LA. Leptomeningeal metastasis of primary central nervous system (CNS) neoplasms. Cancer Treat Res 2005;125:71–85.

88. Niermeijer JM, Somers M, Spliet W, et al. Rapidly progressive coma, hydrocephalus and leukoencephalopathy as presenting features of leptomeningeal metastases. J Neurol 2007;254:1757–8.

89. Wong ET, Joseph JT. Meningeal carcinomatosis in lung cancer. Case 1. Carcinomatous leptomeningeal metastases. J Clin Oncol 2000;18:2926–7.

90. Posner JB. Leptomeningeal metastases. In: Posner JB, editor, Neurologic complications of cancer, vol. 45. Philadelphia: F.A. Davis Co.; 1995. p. 143–71.

91. Wen P. Leptomeningeal metastases. In: Black P, Loeffler J, editors. Cancer of the nervous system. Cambridge: Blackwell Science; 1997. p. 288–309.

92. Grossman SA, Moynihan TJ. Neoplastic meningitis. Neurol Clin 1991;9:843–56.

93. Bruno MK, Raizer J. Leptomeningeal metastases from solid tumors (meningeal carcinomatosis). Cancer Treat Res 2005;125:31–52.

94. Twijnstra A, Ongerboer de Visser BW, van Zanten AP, et al. Serial lumbar and ventricular cerebrospinal fluid biochemical marker measurements in patients with leptomeningeal metastases from solid and hematological tumors. J Neurooncol 1989;7:57–63.

95. Freilich RJ, Krol G, DeAngelis LM. Neuroimaging and cerebrospinal fluid cytology in the diagnosis of leptomeningeal metastasis. Ann Neurol 1995;38:51–7.

96. Mokri B, Parisi JE, Scheithauer BW, et al. Meningeal biopsy in intracranial hypotension: meningeal enhancement on MRI. Neurology 1995;45:1801–7.

97. Rogers LR, Remer SE, Tejwani S. Durable response of breast cancer leptomeningeal metastasis to capecitabine monotherapy. Neuro Oncol 2004;6:63–4.

98. Boogerd W, Dorresteijn LD, van Der Sande JJ, et al. Response of leptomeningeal metastases from breast cancer to hormonal therapy. Neurology 2000;55:117–9.

99. Ozdogan M, Samur M, Bozcuk HS, et al. Durable remission of leptomeningeal metastasis of breast cancer with letrozole: a case report and implications of biomarkers on treatment selection. Jpn J Clin Oncol 2003;33:229–31.

100. Taillibert S, Hildebrand J. Treatment of central nervous system metastases: parenchymal, epidural, and leptomeningeal. Curr Opin Oncol 2006;18:637–43.

101. Mehta M, Bradley K. Radiation therapy for leptomeningeal cancer. Cancer Treat Res 2005;125:147–58.

102. Dalmau J, Rosenfeld MR. Paraneoplastic syndromes of the CNS. Lancet Neurol 2008;7:327–40.

103. Darnell RB, Posner JB. Paraneoplastic syndromes involving the nervous system. N Engl J Med 2003;349:1543–54.

104. Posner JB. Paraneoplastic syndromes. In: Posner JB, editor. Neurologic complications of cancer. Philadelphia: F.A. Davis Co; 1995. p. 353–84.

105. Graus F, Delattre JY, Antoine JC, et al. Recommended diagnostic criteria for paraneoplastic neurological syndromes. J Neurol Neurosurg Psychiatr 2004;75:1135–40.

Optimal Management of Malignant Epidural Spinal Cord Compression

Hai Sun, MD, PhD, Andrew N. Nemecek, MD*

KEYWORDS
- Epidural • Malignant • Management • Neoplasm
- Spinal cord compression

Malignant epidural spinal cord compression (MESCC) is a common complication in patients with advanced neoplasm. This disease occurs when cancer metastasizes to the spine or epidural space and compresses the spinal cord.[1] Patients usually present with acute deterioration of neurologic functions such as inability to ambulate due to the mass effect of the metastatic diseases on the spinal cord. It is of paramount importance that the emergency department (ED) physician appreciate that MESCC is considered a treatable medical emergency, and that prompt management requires swift decision making with the collaboration of specialists such as oncologists, imaging and pathology specialists, and spine surgeons to avoid further deterioration of the patient's neurologic functions.[1–5] The management strategy for MESCC has evolved over the years, in part due to technological advancements in spinal instrumentation. Herein the authors present a primer for the ED team on the epidemiology, pathophysiology, and clinical presentation of MESCC, describe the role of medical and surgical approaches in managing this disease, and, based on recent data, recommend guidelines for use in clinical practice.

EPIDEMIOLOGY

In the United States, approximately 500,000 deaths are attributable to metastatic disease every year. Of all osseous sites, the spinal column is the most common location for metastatic deposits.[6] Almost all major types of systemic cancer can metastasize to the spinal column. Evidence suggests that 2.5% to 5.0% of patients with

A version of this article was previously published in the *Emergency Medicine Clinics of North America*, 27:2.

Department of Neurological Surgery, CH8N, Oregon Health and Science University, 3303 SW Bond Avenue, Portland, OR 97239, USA

* Corresponding author.

E-mail address: nemeceka@ohsu.edu

Hematol Oncol Clin N Am 24 (2010) 537–551

doi:10.1016/j.hoc.2010.03.011

terminal cancers have spinal involvement within the last 2 years of illness, and MESCC occurs in up to 40% of patients who have pre-existing nonspinal metastases.[3–5] The incidence of MESCC varies by primary disease site and patient age. In adults, the most common primary tumor sites leading to MESCC are the prostate, breast, and lung, each accounting for 15% to 20% of all cases. Non-Hodgkin lymphoma, renal cell carcinoma, and multiple myeloma account for 5% to 10%, and the remainder of cases are due to colorectal sarcomas and other unknown primary tumors.[2] In the pediatric population, neuroblastoma, Ewing sarcoma, Wilms tumor, lymphoma, and soft-tissue and bone sarcoma are the most common types that lead to spinal cord compression.[7,8] The most common level of MESCC involvement is the thoracic spine (60%–78%), followed by the lumbar (16%–33%) and cervical spine (4%–15%); multiple levels are involved in up to 50% of patients.[9,10]

PATHOPHYSIOLOGY

The most common way by which a primary malignancy spreads to the spinal column is through direct arterial embolization of tumor cells. Classically, it is believed that the valveless venous system in the spine (Batson's plexus) may facilitate the hematogenous spread of the primary tumor to the spinal column.[11] Recent evidence from animals suggests that arterial embolization may be a more important mechanism for metastasis.[12] This seeding of tumor cells results in an expansive mass in the vertebral body. Compression of the epidural space can be caused by the continued growth and expansion of the mass itself or from retropulsion of bony fragments following collapse of a vertebral body weakened by tumor (**Fig. 1**). Additionally, some tumors, especially lymphoma and neuroblastoma, can reach the epidural space by the direct

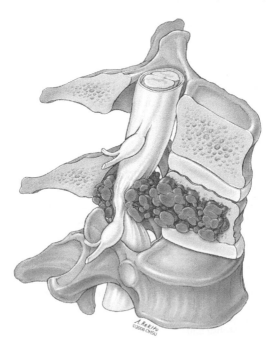

Fig. 1. Metastatic tumor invading the thoracic vertebral body causing circumferential epidural compression of the spinal cord. (*Courtesy of* OHSU Neurological Surgery, Portland, OR; with permission.)

growth of the paravertebral tumor into the spinal canal through an intervertebral foramen.[9] Intramedullary, subdural or lepomeningeal metastases are rarely encountered causes of MESCC.[12]

Animal studies and intraoperative observations have demonstrated that damage to the functional integrity of the spinal cord caused by MESCC is largely due to vascular compromise. First, the tumor mass or bony fragment impinges on the venous plexus surrounding the cord, which results in cord edema. The increased edema causes increased pressure on small arterioles, which leads to diminished capillary blood flow. Disruption of blood flow to the cord leads to white matter ischemia and, with prolonged compression, may eventually cause cord infarction.[13] Production of vascular endothelial growth factor (VEGF) is also associated with spinal cord hypoxia. It has been proposed that steroid efficacy in the treatment of acute MESCC is at least partly due to down-regulation of VEGF expression.[12,14]

Another important mechanism by which metastatic tumors can harm the spinal cord is destabilization of the spinal column. Tumor invasion of the bony spine can lead to failure of the spinal column in the same way as a traumatic injury. Denis proposed a 3-column model for the evaluation of spine stability.[15] In this model (**Fig. 2**), the anterior column is composed of the anterior longitudinal ligament, the anterior annulus, and the anterior portion of the vertebral body. The middle column includes the posterior longitudinal ligament, the posterior annulus, and the posterior portion of the vertebral body. The posterior column includes those spinal structures that are posterior to the posterior longitudinal ligament. Disruption of 2 or 3 columns creates an unstable spine. It has been recognized that it is more common for a malignant lesion to involve the vertebral body and cause it to collapse. Findlay reported, in a small series, that more than half of patients with MESCC had a collapsed vertebral body.[16] Collapse often involved the anterior and middle columns, hence spinal instability.

CLINICAL PRESENTATION

Pretreatment neurologic status is by far the most important predictor of function after treatment.[2,4,6] Therefore, it is highly desirable to diagnose MESCC before the patient develops any neurologic deficits. Most patients with MESCC have a known cancer diagnosis, emphasizing the importance of providing ED personnel with ready access to the prior medical records.

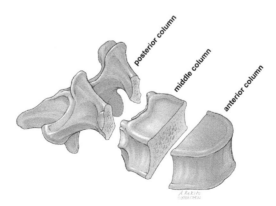

Fig. 2. Denis' 3-column model of spinal stability. Disruption of 2 or 3 columns may lead to structural instability. (*Courtesy of* OHSU Neurological Surgery, Portland, OR; with permission.)

Pain is by far the most common presenting symptom of MESCC, occurring in approximately 83% to 95% of patients. Back pain caused by MESCC can take several forms and local and quality can vary. Initially, pain can be localized and confined to the region of spinal metastases, as the tumor stretches the periosteum or invades adjacent soft tissues. Radicular pain is also common among patients with MESCC and may occur when the tumor mass compresses or invades the nerve roots. Pain is usually worse at night when the patient is recumbent due to lengthening of the spine, or with Valsalva maneuver. A more ominous type of pain is mechanical back pain, which is made worse by movement and partially relieved with rest, may suggest spinal instability caused by vertebral body collapse.[1] This can be a harbinger of subsequent neurologic deterioration. Hence the ED triage team must maintain equipoise when evaluating patients with the common complaint of back pain.

Motor deficit is the second most common symptom of MESCC (60%–85%), followed by sensory deficits (40%–80%). Patient complaints related to these symptoms are often vague. Weakness is frequently described as clumsiness or heaviness which can progress to paralysis. Motor deficit can involve upper and lower motor neurons. Upper motor neuron weakness is more likely to be symmetric, whereas lower motor neuron weakness is often asymmetric and affects the distal end of limbs first.[17,18] Loss of ability to ambulate is usually due to weakness. Sensory deficits rarely occur before motor deficits or pain, and they usually begin distally and ascend as the disease advances.[17,18] Increased susceptibility to falling can indicate the progression of motor and sensory deficits. Autonomic/sphincter dysfunction is typically a later finding (40%–60%).[9,17,19,20] Among elderly patients, urinary retention is a more reliable sign of autonomic sphincter dysfunction than urinary incontinence. Sphincter dysfunction is a poor prognostic indicator for preservation or improvement of ambulatory status.[1]

DIAGNOSIS

A diagnosis of MESCC begins with obtaining a medical history and performing an appropriately focused general physical examination that is coupled with a comprehensive central nervous system (CNS) examination in patients suspected of having MESCC. New onset of back pain or neurologic symptoms such as symmetric weakness or paresthesia in a patient with known cancer should prompt further workup for MESCC. Imaging of the entire spine should be performed on any patient suspected of having MESCC not only to define the diagnosis but also to aid surgical or radiotherapy treatment planning. Magnetic resonance (MR) imaging is currently the gold standard imaging modal for assessing spinal metastatic disease. It is sensitive (93%) and specific (97%) for detection of MESCC [10,11] and because multiple levels are frequently involved, imaging of the entire spine is highly recommended.[21] Conventional computed tomography myelography techniques, with or without MR imaging are used if a patient cannot have MR imaging due to metallic implants.

Other imaging modalities are less useful than MR imaging. Plain films have insufficient sensitivity and specificity to make a diagnosis and they should not be performed; delaying MR imaging should be avoided.[22,23] Radionuclide bone scans and positron emission tomography can detect MESCC but they are not as accurate as MR imaging due to lower resolutions.

MANAGEMENT

Patients with MESCC are usually affected by widespread cancer. Large retrospective studies have reported the median survival time for a patient with MESCC as 3 to 6 months.[4,7] Treatment of spinal metastatic diseases including MESCC is mainly palliative. The goals are to control pain, avoid complications, and preserve neurologic function.

Corticosteroids

Corticosteroids are believed to delay neurologic deterioration by decreasing spinal cord edema and may also have an oncolytic effect on certain tumors, such as lymphoma and multiple myeloma.

As alluded to earlier, the efficacy of corticosteroids in managing patients with MESCC can partially be explained by a role in reduction of hypoxic spinal tissue VEGF expression. In a randomized trial, patients with MESCC were assigned to the treatment arm of a 96-mg intravenous (IV) bolus of dexamethasone followed by 96 mg/d orally for 3 days and a 10-day taper, versus no corticosteroids before radiotherapy. In the group treated with dexamethasone and radiation, ambulatory rates were higher than the group treated with radiation alone at 3 months and 6 months (P<.05).[24]

Although the efficacy of corticosteroids in delaying neurologic deterioration has been proven through these clinical data, the optimal loading and maintenance doses of corticosteroids have not been determined. Studies in animals have found a positive dose-dependent association of dexamethasone's effect in reducing cord edema, which reaches a maximum effect at approximately 100 mg/kg. Vecht and colleagues,[25] in the only randomized trial examining corticosteroid loading dose, reported no difference between an intravenous dexamethasone loading dose of 10 mg versus 100 mg with respect to pain reduction, ambulation, or bladder function. In this trial, the maintenance dose for all patients was 16 mg of oral dexamethasone per day.

Currently, due to lack of consensus, there are 2 widely used dosing regimens for steroids: a high dose (100 mg loading dose, followed by 96 mg/d) and a moderate dose (10 mg loading dose, followed by 16 mg/d). Some physicians advocate using motor symptoms to titrate the steroid dosage; that is, patients with rapidly progressive motor symptoms such as loss of ability to ambulate receive a high dose, whereas patients with minimal or nonprogressive weakness are treated with moderate doses.

Radiation

Palliative radiation therapy has been the standard care for patients with MESCC since the 1950s. The efficacy of radiotherapy in the preservation or improvement of neurologic function in patients with MESCC has been reported in numerous retrospective studies.[4,7,9,26–30] Given a lack of equipoise regarding the efficacy of radiation therapy, a prospective, randomized controlled trial comparing radiation to no radiation would not be ethical. Despite general acceptance of the effectiveness of radiotherapy, the optimal dose and treatment regimen remains controversial. In conventional external-beam fractionated radiotherapy, the proximity of the spinal cord limits the dose that can be delivered. Various dose schedules have been tried for pain relief and reversal of compression. In a systematic review of various dose schedules, Sze and colleagues[31] found no differences in pain relief between single fraction and multifraction radiotherapy. In 1 randomized study, Maranzono and colleagues,[29] reported that a hypofractionation schedule resulted in no difference in back pain relief, maintenance of ambulation, and good bladder function rates among patients with MESCC receiving radiotherapy. In a retrospective study, post-treatment ambulatory rate and motor function improvement were not shown to be affected by the initial dose and number of fractions, but the rate of in-field recurrence was lower with protracted schedules.[30] Because fractionation helps lower the risk of spinal cord injury, the recommendation based on these studies is to give a single fraction of 8 Gy to MESCC patients with limited survival expectations and 3 Gy in 10 fractions to all other patients. Most radiation oncologists adhere to typical schedules of 2.5 to 3.6 Gy delivered in 10 to 15 fractions.

Known predictors of outcome with radiation therapy are: (1) extent of functional limitation at the start of radiation; (2) tumor type; and (3) rapidity of onset of neurologic deficits. For example, 80% to 100% of patients who are still ambulatory when they begin radiation therapy maintain their ability to walk, whereas only one third of patients who are not mobile before treatment regain the ability to walk.[7,30] Primary tumors most sensitive to radiation are lymphoma and seminomatous germ-cell tumor. Most solid tumors, such as breast, prostate, and lung cancers, are considered intermediately radiosensitive. Melanoma, osteosarcoma, and renal cell carcinoma are usually considered to be radioresistant.[32] Although patients with radioresistant tumors may still experience substantial palliation with radiation, the chance of major functional recovery or long-term response to radiation is much less than that for patients with radiosensitive tumors.[7,30] Patients who rapidly develop neurologic deficits are less likely to improve than those who develop deficits more gradually. This may reflect the fact that patients with sudden onset of paralysis have actually suffered an infarction of the spinal cord itself, which is not likely to improve even with relief of the compression. A much weaker predictor of outcome is the extent of subarachnoid block observed on MR imaging; an epidural metastasis that causes minor compression should have a better outcome than a large mass that encircles and deforms the spinal cord, and obliterates the subarachnoid space.[7]

Surgical Treatment

The role of surgical decompression in the management of patients with MESCC has evolved over the years. Historically, radiation alone was the standard treatment for MESCC, largely due to an early study comparing the efficacy of laminectomy followed by radiotherapy with that of radiotherapy alone; no difference in outcome or survival was reported.[9,33] Surgery at that time was a laminectomy that usually did not address the primary site of compression. Laminectomy decompressed the spinal canal and spinal cord but had only been proven to be effective if compression was posterior. As mentioned earlier, MESCC more commonly involves the anterior elements of the spinal column, such as the vertebral body.[16] In the setting of anterior spinal compression, a laminectomy is insufficient to achieve decompression; furthermore, it may lead to loss of spinal stability if the posterior column is disrupted, resulting in neurologic deterioration after surgery. Therefore, this procedure should be reserved for the removal of posterior lesions.

In the 1980s, with the advancement of surgical techniques and spinal instrumentation, it became possible to decompress the spinal cord circumferentially, and reconstruct and immediately stabilize the spine. This procedure can be done by combining an anterior approach, for example, thoracotomy, with a posterior approach, for example, laminectomy and fixation. For the thoracic spine, the most common location of MESCC, a single posterolateral approach can be used. This procedure involves removing anterior compressive lesions, reconstructing the anterior and middle columns of the spine, and restoring the stability of the posterior columns using segmental fixation with pedicle screws and rods (**Figs. 3–6**). A sagittal MR image showing epidural compression of the thoracic spinal cord in a 50-year-old patient with metastatic melanoma and postoperative radiographs of the same patient showing spinal hardware after decompression and stabilization are presented in **Fig. 7**. The advantage of surgical treatment over radiotherapy alone has been

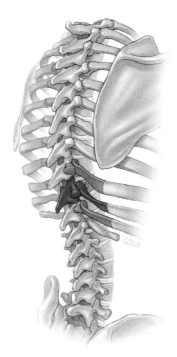

Fig. 3. Area of bony resection for posterolateral approach to anterior and posterior thoracic spinal lesions. (*Courtesy of* OHSU Neurological Surgery, Portland, OR; with permission.)

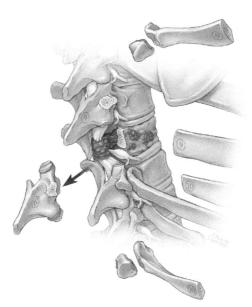

Fig. 4. Posterolateral approach to spinal metastases. T10 lamina, pedicle, and transverse process are removed. T9 and T10 ribs are removed to a distance of 10 cm from the spine, allowing extrapleural dissection and access to the ventral vertebral body. (*Courtesy of* OHSU Neurological Surgery, Portland, OR; with permission.)

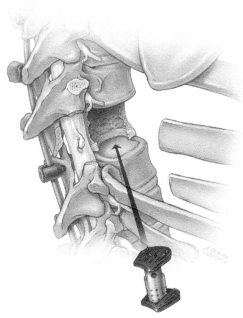

Fig. 5. Pedicle screws and a connecting rod have been placed on the left side to stabilize the spine. The vertebral body and tumor have been resected using a right posterolateral approach, and an expandable titanium cage is then placed into the resection cavity again through a right posterolateral approach, reaching around and under the spinal cord to implant the cage. (*Courtesy of* OHSU Neurological Surgery, Portland, OR; with permission.)

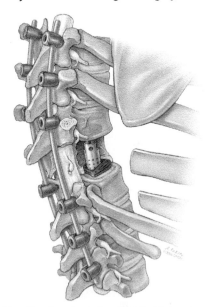

Fig. 6. Final construct. The titanium cage is expanded into place, and screws and rods are placed down the right side. The spine has now been completely decompressed and reconstructed circumferentially though a single posterolateral approach. (*Courtesy of* OHSU Neurological Surgery, Portland, OR; with permission.)

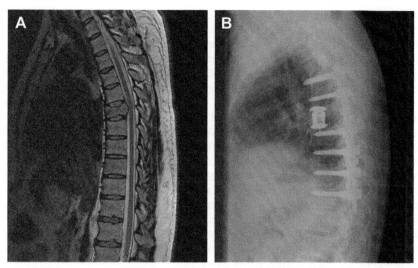

Fig. 7. Illustrative case. Sagittal MR image showing epidural compression of the thoracic spinal cord in a 50-year-old patient with metastatic melanoma (*A*); postoperative radiographs of the same patient showing spinal hardware after decompression and stabilization (*B*). (*Courtesy of* OHSU Neurological Surgery, Portland, OR; with permission.)

suggested in several uncontrolled surgical series.[34–45] In a meta-analysis, Klimo and colleagues[28] reviewed data from 24 surgical articles (999 patients) and 4 radiation articles (543 patients), and reported that surgery followed by radiation leads to higher overall ambulatory success rates than radiation alone (85% vs 64%, $P<.001$).

In 2005, Patchell and colleagues[46] published the first randomized trial that compared direct decompressive and reconstructive surgery followed by postoperative radiotherapy with radiotherapy alone. The study included patients with a known cancer diagnosis, who became symptomatic from MESCC (also demonstrated with MR imaging). All patients in the study were given a loading dose of 100 mg of dexamethasone and then a maintenance dose of 24 mg every 6 hours before being randomly assigned to 1 of the 2 treatment groups. Patients in the radiotherapy alone group received 30 Gy (10 doses of 3 Gy) and the first dose of radiation began within 24 hours of enrollment in the study. Patients in the surgery followed by radiotherapy group were operated on within 24 hours of enrollment in the study and then received radiation within 2 weeks after the surgery. Surgery was performed with the intent of removing as much tumor as possible, and providing immediate decompression and stabilization of the spinal column with the necessary hardware. The primary endpoint of the study was the ability to ambulate after treatment and secondary endpoints included post-treatment continence rates, length of time patients maintained muscle strength, and functional status and survival time. The original study design called for a sample size of 200 patients but the study was stopped early after an interim analysis. One-hundred and one patients were ultimately enrolled in the study over a 10-year period. The percentage of patients able to walk after treatment was significantly ($P = .001$) higher in the surgical group (84%) than in the radiotherapy group (57%). Patients treated with surgery also retained the ability to walk significantly longer than those with radiotherapy alone (median 122 days vs 13 days, $P<.003$). Thirty-two patients (16 in each treatment group) enrolled in the study were unable to walk; a significantly greater proportion of patients in the surgery group regained the ability to walk than patients in the radiation alone group (62% vs 19%, $P = .01$). The need for corticosteroids and opioid analgesics was significantly lower in the surgical group, and muscle strength and functional status were also maintained significantly longer in patients treated with surgery. Survival times were also significantly longer in the surgery group (median, 126 days vs 100 days, $P = .033$). This landmark study confirmed the advantage of a surgical approach in treating MESCC: immediate relief of spinal compression, and stabilization of a diseased and weakened vertebral column.[46] Although this randomized trial clearly established the effectiveness of complex spinal surgery in treating MESCC, the study inclusion criteria prevents the application of data to all patients with this condition. Patients with radiosensitive tumors, neurologic deficits longer than 48 hours, multiple spinal lesions, a mass that compressed only cauda equina or spinal root, and previous radiation treatment were excluded from the study. Given the study limitations, it is incorrect to assume that all patients with MESCC would benefit from surgical treatments. One must consider whether a given patient is medically suitable for surgery. Moreover, if it is unlikely that the patient will live beyond a few weeks or months due to their oncologic disease, it may not be reasonable to perform a surgical procedure that may require several weeks of hospitalization for recovery.

Among the indications for surgical intervention, patient life expectancy is the most difficult to estimate, and the judgment and experience of specialists has been found to be inaccurate.[47–49] Several schemes and a model have been developed to predict the survival of a patient affected by MESCC, however, the predictive values of these systems have been unsatisfactory.[47,48,50,51] In general, many experts believe that factors such as the patient's functional status, the number of metastases in the vertebral body, metastases to the major internal organs (lungs, liver, kidneys, and brain), and the type of primary tumor, all have direct impact on survival. However, an estimate of how these factors influence survival rates remains qualitative.

It is commonly accepted that the goal of direct decompressive surgery is to preserve or recover ambulatory function. In several studies, preoperative ambulatory ability was found to be strongly associated with postoperative ambulation, namely patients who were able to walk before the surgery were likely to retain the ability to walk.[6,34,35,46,52–55] These data suggest that early surgical intervention may benefit patients before ambulatory function begins to decline.

Emerging Treatment Options

Spinal stereotactic radiosurgery (SRS) and other emerging forms of radiotherapy, such as intensity-modulated radiotherapy, allow radiation to be more accurately delivered to the target while minimizing the amount delivered to normal issues. Conventional radiotherapy is typically administered in 10 to 15 fractions with a total radiation dose of 25 to 40 Gy.[30] Stereotactic localization enables multiple radiation beams to converge on the lesion of interest at a high dose, while limiting the exposure of normal tissue. As a result, SRS can be administered in 1 or 2 sessions on an outpatient basis with total dose ranges of 8 to18 Gy. Degen and colleagues,[56] using the CyberKnife frameless robotic radiosurgery system to treat 58 spinal metastatic lesions, reported a significant improvement in pain. Of patients who presented with a neurologic deficit, less than one third improved. The study also demonstrated that SRS produced only mild side effects, maintaining quality of life for the patients. There is a need to test the effectiveness of spinal SRS versus surgery and radiotherapy in the setting of acute MESCC. Shortcomings of SRS include an inability to address the issue of spinal instability and delivery of radiation to large lesions.

Percutaneous vertebroplasty and kyphoplasty have received considerable attention due to their minimal invasiveness. There has been some evidence that these procedures can lead to marked pain relief in patients with intractable pain secondary to pathologic vertebral body fractures.[57] It is to be hoped that these techniques can provide the same pain relief for patients with MESCC when combined with radiotherapy. In an attempt to identify factors predicting ambulatory status after decompressive surgery, Chaichana and colleagues[52] reported that the presence of a pathologic compression fracture on preoperative images was independently associated with postoperative loss of ambulation. This finding prompted the investigators to advocate prompt treatment of metastatic disease before the onset of compression fractures using techniques such as vertebroplasty and kyphoplasty. These treatment options can only be considered if the patient is free of neurologic signs and symptoms caused by vertebral body collapse or tumor extension. The presence of these signs and symptoms is currently considered a relative contraindication for vertebroplasty and kyphoplasty.

Chemotherapy is rarely used in acute management of MESCC because, even with chemosensitive tumors, the response is too slow and unpredictable for it to be effective. In the case of chemosensitive tumors, chemotherapy may be used in conjunction with radiotherapy. Chemotherapy may also be given if a patient who has undergone radiotherapy for cord compression has recurrence and is no longer a candidate for further surgery or radiation.[58,59]

SUMMARY

The management of malignant spinal cord compression has evolved with advances in surgical techniques, chemotherapeutics, and radiation delivery. A growing body of evidence has emerged; including Level I data from a prospective, randomized controlled trial, demonstrating the efficacy of combining surgery with radiation in the treatment of spinal metastases. Clearly, a multidisciplinary approach is necessary to facilitate the management of this oncologic emergency. This approach involves spine surgeons, radiation, and medical oncologists, as well as imaging and pathology specialists. Moreover, the emergency medicine physician is often the "front door" to this multidisciplinary approach. Particularly in cases of previously undiagnosed cancer, it is often the emergency physician who makes the diagnosis and engages the appropriate specialists.

Patients with malignancy who present with new onset of neurologic signs and symptoms should undergo emergent evaluation including MR imaging of the entire spine. If MESCC is diagnosed, patients should receive an intravenous loading dose of 10 mg dexamethasone followed by a maintenance dose of 4 to 6 mg (intravenous or oral) every 6 to 8 hours. Simultaneously, the spine surgery and oncology teams should be immediately consulted. If indicated, patients should undergo maximal tumor resection and stabilization, followed by postoperative radiotherapy administered in 10 to 15 fractions with a total radiation dose of 25 to 40 Gy. In patients for whom surgery is contraindicated, palliative radiotherapy still remains the standard of care. Emerging treatment options such as stereotactic radiosurgery and vertebroplasty may be able to provide some symptomatic relief for patients who cannot undergo surgery.

ACKNOWLEDGMENTS

The authors would like to express their appreciation and thanks to Shirley McCartney, PhD, for editorial assistance, and Andy Rekito, MS, for assistance with digital illustrations.

REFERENCES

1. Cole JS, Patchell RA. Metastatic epidural spinal cord compression. Lancet Neurol 2008;7:459–66.
2. Bach F, Larsen BH, Rohde K, et al. Metastatic spinal cord compression. Occurrence, symptoms, clinical presentations and prognosis in 398 patients with spinal cord compression. Acta Neurochir 1990;107:37–43.
3. Byrne TN. Spinal cord compression from epidural metastases [see comment]. N Engl J Med 1992;327:614–9.
4. Loblaw DA, Laperriere NJ, Mackillop WJ. A population-based study of malignant spinal cord compression in Ontario. Clin Oncol (R Coll Radiol) 2003;15: 211–7.
5. Quinn JA, DeAngelis LM. Neurologic emergencies in the cancer patient. Semin Oncol 2000;27:311–21.
6. Aaron AD. The management of cancer metastatic to bone. JAMA 1994;272: 1206–9.
7. Helweg-Larsen S, Sorensen PS, Kreiner S. Prognostic factors in metastatic spinal cord compression: a prospective study using multivariate analysis of variables influencing survival and gait function in 153 patients. Int J Radiat Oncol Biol Phys 2000;46:1163–9.
8. Raffel C, Neave VC, Lavine S, et al. Treatment of spinal cord compression by epidural malignancy in childhood. Neurosurgery 1991;28:349–52.
9. Gilbert RW, Kim JH, Posner JB. Epidural spinal cord compression from metastatic tumor: diagnosis and treatment. Ann Neurol 1978;3:40–51.
10. Schiff D, O'Neill BP, Wang CH, et al. Neuroimaging and treatment implications of patients with multiple epidural spinal metastases. Cancer 1998;83:1593–601.
11. Li KC, Poon PY. Sensitivity and specificity of MRI in detecting malignant spinal cord compression and in distinguishing malignant from benign compression fractures of vertebrae. Magn Reson Imaging 1988;6:547–56.
12. Arguello F, Baggs RB, Duerst RE, et al. Pathogenesis of vertebral metastasis and epidural spinal cord compression. Cancer 1990;65:98–106.
13. Siegal T. Spinal cord compression: from laboratory to clinic. Eur J Cancer 1995; 31A:1748–53.
14. Benton RL, Whittemore SR. VEGF165 therapy exacerbates secondary damage following spinal cord injury. Neurochem Res 2003;28:1693–703.
15. Denis F. The three column spine and its significance in the classification of acute thoracolumbar spinal injuries. Spine 1983;8:817–31.
16. Findlay GF. The role of vertebral body collapse in the management of malignant spinal cord compression. J Neurol Neurosurg Psychiatr 1987;50:151–4.
17. Heldmann U, Myschetzky PS, Thomsen HS. Frequency of unexpected multifocal metastasis in patients with acute spinal cord compression. Evaluation by low-field MR imaging in cancer patients. Acta Radiol 1997;38:372–5.
18. Helweg-Larsen S, Sorensen PS. Symptoms and signs in metastatic spinal cord compression: a study of progression from first symptom until diagnosis in 153 patients. Eur J Cancer 1994;30A:396–8.
19. Martenson JA Jr, Evans RG, Lie MR, et al. Treatment outcome and complications in patients treated for malignant epidural spinal cord compression (SCC). J Neurooncol 1985;3:77–84.
20. Torma T. Malignant tumors of the spine and spinal epidural space: a study based on 250 histologically verified cases. Acta Chir Scand Suppl 1957;225: 1–176.

21. Loughrey GJ, Collins CD, Todd SM, et al. Magnetic resonance imaging in the management of suspected spinal canal disease in patients with known malignancy. Clin Radiol 2000;55:849–55.

22. Kienstra GE, Terwee CB, Dekker FW, et al. Prediction of spinal epidural metastases. Arch Neurol 2000;57:690–5.

23. Ruckdeschel JC. Early detection and treatment of spinal cord compression. Oncology (Williston Park) 2005;19:81–6 [discussion: 86].

24. Sorensen S, Helweg-Larsen S, Mouridsen H, et al. Effect of high-dose dexamethasone in carcinomatous metastatic spinal cord compression treated with radiotherapy: a randomised trial. Eur J Cancer 1994;30A:22–7.

25. Vecht CJ, Haaxma-Reiche H, van Putten WL, et al. Initial bolus of conventional versus high-dose dexamethasone in metastatic spinal cord compression. Neurology 1989;39:1255–7.

26. Barron KD, Hirano A, Araki S, et al. Experiences with metastatic neoplasms involving the spinal cord. Neurology 1959;9:91–106.

27. Constans JP, de Divitiis E, Donzelli R, et al. Spinal metastases with neurological manifestations. Review of 600 cases. J Neurosurg 1983;59:111–8.

28. Klimo P Jr, Thompson CJ, Kestle JR, et al. A meta-analysis of surgery versus conventional radiotherapy for the treatment of metastatic spinal epidural disease. Neuro Oncol 2005;7:64–76.

29. Maranzano E, Bellavita R, Rossi R, et al. Short-course versus split-course radiotherapy in metastatic spinal cord compression: results of a phase III, randomized, multicenter trial [see comment]. J Clin Oncol 2005;23:3358–65.

30. Rades D, Stalpers LJ, Veninga T, et al. Evaluation of five radiation schedules and prognostic factors for metastatic spinal cord compression. J Clin Oncol 2005;23:3366–75.

31. Sze WM, Shelley MD, Held I, et al. Palliation of metastatic bone pain: single fraction versus multifraction radiotherapy—a systematic review of randomised trials [see comment]. Clin Oncol (R Coll Radiol) 2003;15:345–52.

32. Peters LJ. The ESTRO Regaud lecture. Inherent radiosensitivity of tumor and normal tissue cells as a predictor of human tumor response. Radiother Oncol 1990;17:177–90.

33. Greenberg HS, Kim JH, Posner JB. Epidural spinal cord compression from metastatic tumor: results with a new treatment protocol. Ann Neurol 1980;8:361–6.

34. Fourney DR, Abi-Said D, Lang FF, et al. Use of pedicle screw fixation in the management of malignant spinal disease: experience in 100 consecutive procedures. J Neurosurg 2001;94:25–37.

35. Gokaslan ZL, York JE, Walsh GL, et al. Transthoracic vertebrectomy for metastatic spinal tumors. J Neurosurg 1998;89:599–609.

36. Harrington KD. Anterior cord decompression and spinal stabilization for patients with metastatic lesions of the spine. J Neurosurg 1984;61:107–17.

37. Hosono N, Yonenobu K, Fuji T, et al. Vertebral body replacement with a ceramic prosthesis for metastatic spinal tumors. Spine 1995;20:2454–62.

38. North RB, LaRocca VR, Schwartz J, et al. Surgical management of spinal metastases: analysis of prognostic factors during a 10-year experience. J Neurosurg Spine 2005;2:564–73.

39. Overby MC, Rothman AS. Anterolateral decompression for metastatic epidural spinal cord tumors. Results of a modified costotransversectomy approach. J Neurosurg 1985;62:344–8.

40. Siegal T, Siegal T, Robin G, et al. Anterior decompression of the spine for metastatic epidural cord compression: a promising avenue of therapy? Ann Neurol 1982;11:28–34.

41. Siegal T, Tiqva P, Siegal T. Vertebral body resection for epidural compression by malignant tumors. Results of forty-seven consecutive operative procedures. J Bone Joint Surg Am 1985;67:375–82.

42. Sundaresan N, Galicich JH, Bains MS, et al. Vertebral body resection in the treatment of cancer involving the spine. Cancer 1984;53:1393–6.

43. Wang JC, Boland P, Mitra N, et al. Single-stage posterolateral transpedicular approach for resection of epidural metastatic spine tumors involving the vertebral body with circumferential reconstruction: results in 140 patients. Invited submission from the Joint Section Meeting on Disorders of the Spine and Peripheral Nerves, March 2004. J Neurosurg Spine 2004;1:287–98.

44. Weigel B, Maghsudi M, Neumann C, et al. Surgical management of symptomatic spinal metastases. Postoperative outcome and quality of life. Spine 1999;24:2240–6.

45. Young RF, Post EM, King GA. Treatment of spinal epidural metastases. Randomized prospective comparison of laminectomy and radiotherapy. J Neurosurg 1980;53:741–8.

46. Patchell RA, Tibbs PA, Regine WF, et al. Direct decompressive surgical resection in the treatment of spinal cord compression caused by metastatic cancer: a randomised trial [see comment]. Lancet 2005;366:643–8.

47. Tokuhashi Y, Matsuzaki H, Toriyama S, et al. Scoring system for the preoperative evaluation of metastatic spine tumor prognosis [see comment]. Spine 1990;15:1110–3.

48. Tomita K, Kawahara N, Kobayashi T, et al. Surgical strategy for spinal metastases [see comment]. Spine 2001;26:298–306.

49. van der Linden YM, Dijkstra SP, Vonk EJ, et al. Prediction of survival in patients with metastases in the spinal column: results based on a randomized trial of radiotherapy. Cancer 2005;103:320–8.

50. Bartels RH, Feuth T, van der Maazen R, et al. Development of a model with which to predict the life expectancy of patients with spinal epidural metastasis. Cancer 2007;110:2042–9.

51. Tokuhashi Y, Matsuzaki H, Oda H, et al. A revised scoring system for preoperative evaluation of metastatic spine tumor prognosis. Spine 2005;30:2186–91.

52. Chaichana KL, Woodworth GF, Sciubba DM, et al. Predictors of ambulatory function after decompressive surgery for metastatic epidural spinal cord compression. Neurosurgery 2008;62:683–92 [discussion: 683–92].

53. Jackson RJ, Loh SC, Gokaslan ZL. Metastatic renal cell carcinoma of the spine: surgical treatment and results [erratum appears in J Neurosurg 2001 Apr;94(2 Suppl):340]. J Neurosurg 2001;94:18–24.

54. Ogihara S, Seichi A, Hozumi T, et al. Prognostic factors for patients with spinal metastases from lung cancer [see comment]. Spine 2006;31:1585–90.

55. Sciubba DM, Gokaslan ZL. Diagnosis and management of metastatic spine disease. Surg Oncol 2006;15:141–51.

56. Degen JW, Gagnon GJ, Voyadzis JM, et al. CyberKnife stereotactic radiosurgical treatment of spinal tumors for pain control and quality of life. J Neurosurg Spine 2005;2:540–9.

57. Fourney DR, Schomer DF, Nader R, et al. Percutaneous vertebroplasty and kyphoplasty for painful vertebral body fractures in cancer patients. J Neurosurg 2003;98:21–30.

58. Boogerd W, van der Sande JJ, Kroger R, et al. Effective systemic therapy for spinal epidural metastases from breast carcinoma. Eur J Cancer Clin Oncol 1989;25:149–53.
59. Sinoff CL, Blumsohn A. Spinal cord compression in myelomatosis: response to chemotherapy alone. Eur J Cancer Clin Oncol 1989;25:197–200.

Electrolyte Complications of Malignancy

Robert F. Kacprowicz, MD[a,b,c,*], Jeremy D. Lloyd, MD[a,c]

KEYWORDS

- Malignancy • Electrolytes • Hypoglycemia • Hyponatremia
- Hypercalcemia • Hyperphosphatemia

Electrolyte abnormalities are perhaps the most common laboratory finding in patients with malignancies who present to the emergency department. Although most minor abnormalities have no specific treatment, severe clinical manifestations of several notable electrolytes occur with significant frequency in the setting of malignancy. If improperly treated, abnormalities of serum sodium, glucose, calcium, magnesium, and phosphorus may have serious consequences. A review of the most serious electrolyte abnormalities associated with malignancy follows.

HYPONATREMIA

Hyponatremia is a common electrolyte disorder, reported to occur in 3.8% of emergency department patients.[1] Among the population of emergency department patients with underlying malignancy, hyponatremia occurs most commonly with small cell lung cancers. Hyponatremia has been reported with other malignancies, including primary and metastatic malignancies of the brain, pancreatic adenocarcinoma, and prostate cancer.[2] Hyponatremia has also been reported in association with treatment with chemotherapeutic agents, particularly cisplatin and carboplatin.[3] Regardless of the associated malignancy, hyponatremia can present as either an incidental finding or with life-threatening severity. Correction of hyponatremia requires an understanding

A version of this article was previously published in the *Emergency Medicine Clinics of North America*, 27:2.

[a] San Antonio Uniformed Services Health Education Consortium Residency in Emergency Medicine, San Antonio, TX, USA

[b] Department of Emergency Medicine, University of New Mexico School of Medicine, Albuquerque, NM, USA

[c] Department of Emergency Medicine, Wilford Hall USAF Medical Center, 2200 Bergquist Drive Suite 1/59 EMDS, Lackland AFB, TX 78236, USA

* Corresponding author. Department of Emergency Medicine, Wilford Hall USAF Medical Center, 2200 Bergquist Drive Suite 1/59 EMDS, Lackland AFB, TX 78236.

E-mail address: robert.kacprowicz@lackland.af.mil

of both the rapidity with which the hyponatremia has developed as well as the potential complications of treatment.

Pathophysiology

Syndrome of inappropriate antidiuretic hormone

Hyponatremia associated with malignancy is most commonly caused by the syndrome of inappropriate antidiuretic hormone (SIADH) secretion. Ectopic secretion of arginine vasopressin (AVP) by tumor cells appears to play a significant role in the development of hyponatremia.[4] Small cell lung cancer is particularly notorious for elevated levels of circulating AVP despite serum hypotonicity.[4] Other hormones have been implicated in the pathogenesis of hyponatremia of malignancy, including atrial natriuretic peptide, but their ultimate contribution to hyponatremia remains somewhat unclear.[5]

Elevated levels of AVP in patients with malignancy cause hyponatremia primarily due to inappropriate retention of free water at the collecting-duct level despite relative serum hypotonicity.[6] Normally in the setting of hypotonicity, the secretion of AVP is suppressed. In malignancy, the release of AVP by tumor cells does not respond to changes in serum tonicity, and, as a result, AVP remains present in the circulation and results in cyclic AMP-mediated insertion of water channels in the collecting ducts (aquaporin 2).[7] The absorption of free water at the collecting-duct level results in worsening hypotonicity and inappropriately concentrated urine.[7] Clinically, the result is hyponatremia in an apparently euvolemic patient.

Renal salt wasting

Hyponatremia of malignancy has also been reported as a complication of chemotherapy. Both cisplatin and carboplatin have been reported to cause hyponatremia.[3] The mechanism for hyponatremia associated with chemotherapeutic drugs is believed to be renal salt wasting syndrome (RSWS). In this disease process, damage to the renal tubules with subsequent inability to retain sodium is thought to result in increased sodium loss.[8] Clinically, the patient will appear hyponatremic with euvolemia; however, the treatment of RSWS is sodium supplementation rather than water restriction. An elevated spot urine sodium level may suggest RSWS. In SIADH, urinary excretion of sodium is usually normal or decreased. Definitive diagnosis of RSWS, however, can only be made after measurement of daily sodium intake and excretion. RSWS is diagnosed when daily sodium intake is less than urinary excretion.[3] In extremis, however, treatment of hyponatremia due to RSWS is identical to the treatment of hyponatremia due to SIADH.

Clinical Manifestations

The clinical presentation of hyponatremia is largely related to the acuity with which the sodium has declined and has less direct correlation with the actual measured sodium. Levels of decline greater than 0.5 mEq/L/h appear to be more likely to result in serious sequelae, but considerable variation exists between individuals.[9] Most symptomatic individuals will have serum sodium less than 120 mEq/L; however, symptoms have been reported with sodium levels of 129 mEq/L or less.[7]

The brain appears to be the organ most sensitive to changes in the serum sodium level. If the rate of sodium decline outstrips the adaptive capabilities of the brain, symptoms of hyponatremia develop. When the rate of sodium decline is slower, the brain will adapt by expelling potassium and other osmotically active substances (osmolytes) to maintain normal cell volume. These osmolytes include amino acids, myoinositol, creatine, and creatine phosphate.[7] If, however, the rate of sodium decline exceeds the rate at which the brain can expel osmolytes, water shifts intracellularly down the osmotic gradient and results in cerebral edema.

In the setting of acute hyponatremia, the manifestations of the resultant cerebral edema may be severe and commonly include nausea, vomiting, headaches, seizures, coma, and respiratory arrest as the brain progressively swells. Increased intracranial pressure may eventually result in death due to herniation if hyponatremia is not treated.[10]

If hyponatremia develops more slowly, the symptoms may be less severe but present nonetheless. In the patient with chronic hyponatremia, brain cells have had more time to expel osmolytes and maintain near-normal cell volumes. Patients with chronic hyponatremia appear to be at very low risk of life-threatening cerebral edema and present with more subtle symptoms of brain dysfunction.[11] If the level of hyponatremia becomes severe (<120), seizures and altered mental status may still be present, and the sodium will require judicious correction.

In the emergency department, frequently, it will not be possible to determine the acuity of the hyponatremia. In the vast majority of out-of-hospital acquired cases of severe hyponatremia, the hyponatremia is chronic, and particular attention must be paid to the treatment of these patients, as they appear to be at much higher risk of treatment-related severe complications, particularly osmotic demyelination syndrome (ODS).[12] Rapidly correcting the sodium of a patient with chronic hyponatremia and minimal symptoms can be disastrous, so the decision to aggressively treat the hyponatremia should be made with a careful assessment of the risks and benefits of therapy.

OSMOTIC DEMYELINATION SYNDROME

The most feared complication of the treatment of hyponatremia is the ODS, previously known as central pontine myelinolysis. ODS was first reported in 1959 as a consequence of the treatment of a severely hyponatremic alcoholic patient.[13] Histologically, ODS is characterized by the destruction of oligodendrocytes and myelin in the central portion of the pons as well as the basal ganglia and cerebellum.[14] The clinical presentation of patients who develop ODS as a consequence of treatment of hyponatremia includes quadriparesis or quadriplegia, pseudobulbar palsy, and altered mental status. In the worst cases, patients develop the "locked-in syndrome," coma, and death days after treatment for hyponatremia.[15]

The pathophysiology of ODS is complex but appears to be related to brain cell shrinkage and concentrated ion damage during rapid changes in serum tonicity. As described previously, the response to chronic hyponatremia is the release of organic osmolytes from neurons. This adaptive response is protective in the setting of long-standing hyponatremia.[16] During acute correction, however, susceptible areas of the brain appear to be less able to reaccumulate these essential osmolytes.[17] In humans, areas less able to react to osmotic stress appear to be the neurons of the central pons, basal ganglia, and areas of the cerebellum, resulting in the potentially devastating constellation of neurologic findings seen in ODS.

ODS appears to be related to both the severity and the chronicity of hyponatremia. Chronic severe hyponatremia presents the greatest risk for development of ODS with rapid correction of the serum sodium. Most cases of ODS have been reported in patients with chronic hyponatremia of less than 120 mEq/L.[18] In the setting of malnutrition, however, ODS has been reported with higher serum sodium levels, a fact of significance in the treatment of hyponatremic cancer patients who are also at risk for malnutrition due to cachexia.[19]

The development of ODS also appears to be directly related to the rate of rise of the serum sodium. Rates greater than 12 mEq/L/24 h are strongly associated with the development of ODS.[11] Others have reported ODS occurring with rates of correction as low as 8 mEq/L/24 h, and the most recent consensus guidelines recommend limiting correction of the serum sodium to 8 mEq/L/24 h to avoid ODS.[6]

Treatment

Rapidly correcting the sodium of a patient with chronic hyponatremia and minimal symptoms can be disastrous, so the decision to aggressively treat the hyponatremia should be made with a careful assessment of the risks and benefits of therapy. In the emergency department, patients with altered mental status, seizures, respiratory depression, or coma require emergent correction of hyponatremia. If symptoms are milder, the risk of rapid correction of hyponatremia causing ODS generally outweighs the benefits, and these patients should be treated with simple fluid restriction.[6]

If the decision is made to correct hyponatremia emergently, the current treatment of choice is 3% saline infusion. Numerous formulas have been described for the calculation of free water excess, sodium deficit, and so on, but these formulas are cumbersome to use and not entirely reliable. A simpler approach is to infuse 1 cm^3/kg body weight of 3% NS per hour, which will result in an increase of 1 mEq/L serum sodium per hour.[6] Rates as high as 2 to 4 cm^3/kg/h can be tolerated in the short term when symptoms require, but in any case, treatment should be halted once one of three end points is reached:[1] resolution of symptoms,[2] serum sodium of 120 mEq/L is reached, or the daily limit of 8 mEq/L correction is reached.[6,12] Of course, hourly monitoring of the serum sodium is mandatory to prevent overcorrection.

In the event overcorrection does occur, relowering of the serum sodium through the infusion of D5W has the potential to reduce the risk of ODS and should be considered.[20]

If the patient experiences seizures, standard antiepileptic treatment should be used in addition to correction of the hyponatremia with hypertonic saline. Patients at risk for volume overload or with a history of congestive heart failure may be given 20 to 40 mg of furosemide to enhance diuresis.[6]

Disposition

Admission is warranted for any patient with significant symptoms due to hyponatremia. In the patient without symptoms, admission for fluid restriction and further evaluation is generally warranted if the serum sodium is at or less than 125 mEq/L, because symptoms most commonly develop below this level.[10] In the intermediate range (126–130 mEq/L), disposition should be based on the availability of expeditious follow-up care.

Future Directions

A new class of medications, arginine vasopressin receptor (AVPR) antagonists (vaptans), has recently been approved for clinical use and holds significant promise for future treatment of hyponatremia.[6] This is particularly true in cases of malignancy-associated SIADH, as the mechanism of action of these drugs would seem to be perfectly designed to counteract the effects of tumor-associated elevation of circulating AVP at the renal collecting-duct level. By interacting directly with the vasopressin receptor, AVPR antagonists cause an almost pure aquaresis by inhibiting the insertion of aquaporin 2 channels into the collecting duct and, thereby, result in a relative increase in serum sodium at the expense of free water diuresis.[21]

Several studies have demonstrated the usefulness of AVPR antagonists in euvolemic and hypervolemic hyponatremia.[22,23] The only AVPR antagonist currently approved for use is conivaptan, which has been approved for use in hospitalized patients with euvolemic hyponatremia due to SIADH, adrenal insufficiency, and hypothyroidism.[24]

Conivaptan is given as an intravenous (IV) bolus of 20 mg over 30 minutes and then by continuous infusion of 20 to 40 mg over the next 24 hours.[24] Side effects due to conivaptan have reportedly been mild and most commonly include orthostatic dizziness, headache, and nausea.[23] Apart from a higher level of orthostatic dizziness in the treated patients, other side effects are comparable to those with placebo.[23]

The average increase in serum sodium in patients receiving vaptans in clinical trials has been 8 mEq/L, well within the safety range recommended for correction of hyponatremia to prevent ODS.[25] Nine percent of patients had excessive rates of correction of sodium, but no cases of ODS have been reported thus far.[24]

No clinical trials have specifically addressed the use of vaptans for the treatment of severely symptomatic hyponatremia, either alone or as an adjunct to the use of hypertonic saline. Therefore, the use of vaptans in the emergency department, although enticing, cannot be currently recommended for the treatment of symptomatic hyponatremia related to malignancy.

HYPOGLYCEMIA OF MALIGNANCY

Tumor-associated hypoglycemia is a relatively rare complication of malignancy. Hypoglycemia of malignancy has been described in association with 3 main etiologies. The most common cause is nonislet cell tumor hypoglycemia (NICTH).[26] Second, but perhaps more well known, is hypoglycemia due to insulin secretion by islet cell tumors of the pancreas.[27] Finally, end-stage metastatic carcinoma of nearly any source that has heavily infiltrated the liver or adrenal glands may cause hypoglycemia.[28] In the emergency department, the diagnosis and treatment of tumor-associated hypoglycemia requires careful evaluation for other possible causes of hypoglycemia. When other causes have been excluded, treatment of tumor-associated hypoglycemia may be curative or palliative.

Pathophysiology

Perhaps the most well known cause of tumor-associated hypoglycemia is the insulinoma of the pancreas. Insulinoma is a well-known but relatively rare tumor, occurring with an incidence of 1 to 4 per million people.[27] About 90% of insulinomas are benign, and surgical treatment is curative.[29] Insulinomas almost exclusively occur in the pancreas and represent deregulated production of insulin by beta cell tumors.[30]

In the case of NICTH, hypoglycemia is associated with a variety of tumors, including those of mesenchymal, epithelial, and hematopoietic origin.[29] The most common tumors among these tend to be fibrosarcomas, mesotheliomas, leiomyosarcomas, hepatomas, lung cancers, as well as gastric and pancreatic exocrine tumors.[29] NICTH appears to be caused by the secretion of insulin-like growth factor II, a circulating hormone normally synthesized in the liver, which is capable of activating insulin receptors and resulting in hypoglycemia.[31]

In the final instance, that of metastatic malignancy infiltrating the liver or adrenal glands, hypoglycemia is thought to occur either due to simple tissue destruction or due to as yet not fully identified secondary mechanisms, including secretion of tumor necrosis factor alpha, interleukins 1 and 6, or other mechanisms.[30] Research in animals tends to favor the latter explanation, as all of these compounds have been shown to cause profound hypoglycemia.[30]

Clinical Manifestations

Tumor-associated hypoglycemia presents no differently from hypoglycemia due to other mechanisms and should be suspected in any cancer patient with altered level of consciousness, obtundation, or bizarre behavior.[32]

Given the rarity of this disorder, however, a dedicated search for other causes of hypoglycemia should be undertaken before ascribing the symptoms and glucose level to tumor origin. If the patient is diabetic, effort must be taken to evaluate oral intake as well as medication regimen. A complete evaluation for infection or other organ dysfunction may also be warranted, because sepsis, renal failure, and liver failure are all well known, and more common, causes of hypoglycemia in the acutely ill emergency department patient.[29] In the absence of diabetes, infection, or organ dysfunction, evaluation for surreptitious use of insulin or other hypoglycemic agents should also be undertaken, because that is likely the most common cause of hypoglycemia in nondiabetics.[29]

When the patient is not known to have cancer, the diagnosis of tumor-associated hypoglycemia may be particularly difficult. Patients who are ultimately diagnosed with tumor-associated hypoglycemia have frequently suffered from long-standing bouts of recurrent fasting hypoglycemia without an identifiable cause. Admission for further evaluation of any patient with recurrent hypoglycemia with no identifiable cause is warranted, as evaluation of insulin, C-peptide and insulin-like growth factor I and II levels may be very helpful in elucidating the cause and expediting the further workup of suspected tumor-associated hypoglycemia.[26]

Treatment

Once hypoglycemia has been identified, the initial treatment is with glucose and glucose-containing solutions via standard regimens, followed by feeding once consciousness is normalized.

After the acute episode, treatment is directed at either curative or palliative measures. In the case of insulinomas and nonmetastatic tumors causing NICTH, surgical excision may be curative.[30] If operative treatment is not possible due to coexisting disease, invasive disease, and/or metastatic disease, treatment in concert with an endocrinologist may provide relief from symptomatic hypoglycemia. Depending on the tumor, regimens composed of prednisone with or without somatostatin analogs appear to be effective in eliminating the occurrence of symptomatic hypoglycemia.[26]

Disposition

As discussed above, admission is warranted for any patient with hypoglycemia that is recurrent or for which no readily reversible cause can be found (eg, diabetic who has skipped a meal). This is particularly true of those in whom a diagnosis of tumor-associated hypoglycemia has not been made as expedited workup and surgical treatment may be curative.

In the case of a patient with known insulinoma, NICTH, or metastatic malignancy, the ultimate disposition decision should be made in concert with the patient, the patient's oncologist, and likely in consultation with an endocrinologist.

HYPERCALCEMIA

Hypercalcemia is the most common serious electrolyte abnormality in adults with malignancies. It has been reported to occur in 20% to 40% of patients during their disease.[33] The presence of hypercalcemia associated with cancer is associated with a poor prognosis, as this metabolic disorder may result in numerous life-threatening complications, including severe dehydration, bradycardia, seizures, pancreatitis, and coma. Up to 50% of patients die within 30 days of detection of elevated calcium levels.[34]

Pathophysiology

Hypercalcemia typically complicates cancers of the breast, lung, head, and neck as well as leukemia and multiple myeloma. There appears to be a complex set of interactions between bone synthesis and degradation that is responsible for the elevated calcium. Contrary to expectations, bone metastasis does not seem to be required. In patients with hypercalcemia and squamous cell carcinoma of the lung, only 16% have bone lesions, whereas patients with numerous bony metastases from small cell carcinoma of the lung rarely have hypercalcemia.[35]

Four mechanisms have been described to be responsible for hypercalcemia associated with malignancy. Local osteolytic hypercalcemia, comprising 20% of cases, results from significant increase in osteoclastic bone resorption in areas surrounding malignant cells within marrow space. The most common type of hypercalcemia associated with cancer is referred to as humoral hypercalcemia of malignancy (HHM), responsible for 80% of the cases. It is primarily caused by the secretion of humoral factors from tumor cells. Parathyroid hormone-related peptide is the major humoral factor responsible for the elevated serum calcium. This peptide increases bone resorption and decreases renal calcium excretion. Hodgkin's disease, non-Hodgkin's lymphoma, myeloma, and some solid tumors secrete the active form of Vitamin D, 1,25-dihydroxyvitamin D (1,25(OH)2D), causing hypercalcemia due to enhanced intestinal absorption of calcium and increased osteoclastic bone resorption. Finally, there are rare reports of hypercalcemia due to ectopic secretion of PTH by tumors such as ovarian carcinoma.[36,37]

Calcium exists in the extracellular state in a free ionized form or bound to other molecules. The typical laboratory value for total calcium ranges from 8.5 to 10.5 mg/dL. Only about 45% of the total calcium is biologically active in the ionized form. Therefore, laboratory measurement of total calcium can be misleading, since the serum albumin level significantly influences it. Mathematical formulas correcting for albumin have proven to be inaccurate.[38] Since many patients with advanced malignancy will be hypoalbuminemic, an ionized calcium level should be measured if available.

Clinical Manifestations

Hypercalcemia of malignancy typically presents with nonspecific signs and symptoms. The emergency physician must consider calcium abnormalities in any cancer patient with mental status changes or lethargy. In general, calcium levels do not correlate with symptoms, since the acuity of the rise is more important. Hypercalcemia associated with cancer normally occurs rapidly and, therefore, the symptoms of hypercalcemia are more dramatic. The patients suffer from severe dehydration, nausea, vomiting, confusion, and stupor. Patients with more chronic hypercalcemia will complain of anorexia, nausea, vomiting, constipation, polydipsia, polyuria, and memory loss.[39]

Gastrointestinal symptoms, such as nausea, vomiting, anorexia, and constipation, result from smooth muscle relaxation. Neurologically patients may be lethargic, hypotonic, confused, or comatose. The elevated calcium can cause polyuria, nephrolithiasis, and dehydration. The dehydration can exacerbate the hypercalcemia by renal efforts to expand volume through proximal tubule resorption of sodium and calcium. The calcium can also directly affect the electric conduction pathways of the heart. Electrocardiogram features include shortened heart-rate corrected QT intervals, broadened T waves, and first-degree atrioventricular block.

Since hypercalcemia presents in advanced tumors, the malignancy will be evident on presentation, and as mentioned earlier, prognosis is poor. Breast carcinoma and multiple myeloma are the exceptions, as they may typically be successfully treated in the hypercalcemic patient. Successful urgent treatment of the elevated calcium allows time to treat the underlying malignancy and may ultimately result in long-term survival for the patient.

Treatment

Efforts to rapidly lower serum calcium levels in the severely hypercalcemic patient should be made alongside efforts to reverse complications and identify the underlying cause. The most common cause for hypercalcemia in the ED, primary hyperparathyroidism, can be confirmed by elevated PTH level. In contrast, hypercalcemia associated with malignancy will have a low to normal PTH level except for the rare cases due to ectopic production of PTH. Overall management of the hypercalcemic patient should be considered in the context of the underlying disease and clinical condition. Treatment should focus on improving quality of life, mental status, and kidney function and allow for effective therapy. The physician should also note that in certain situations, such as when no improvement in quality of life can be expected and pain control is difficult, the effects of hypercalcemia might provide relief in the dying patient with advanced metastatic disease.

Basic strategies for lowering calcium levels in mild cases focus on decreasing calcium intake and increasing mobility of the patient. Calcium should be removed from parenteral feedings and any oral supplementation stopped. Any other medications that may lead to high calcium levels, such as lithium, vitamin D, thiazides, or calcitriol should also be discontinued. A consideration of reduction in sedatives and analgesics, which may lead to increased weight-bearing mobility, will also be beneficial.

More aggressive therapy is required for successful treatment of severe hypercalcemia (>14 mg/dL) (**Table 1**). Patients are typically profoundly dehydrated; therefore, initial treatment should begin with volume expansion. Recommendations call for IV hydration with normal saline at 200 to 500 mL/h. Volume expansion increases calcium excretion by decreasing passive reabsorption in the proximal tubule and the loop of Henle. Once dehydration is corrected and adequate urine output is achieved, a loop

Table 1 Treatment for severe hypercalcemia		
Therapy	**Dosing**	**Frequency**
Rehydration	200–500 mL/h of 0.9% NaCl	Qd x 1–5 d
Furosemide	20–40 mg IV (after hydration)	Q12–24 h
Pamidronate	60–90 mg IV over 2–4 h	Once
Zoledronate	4 mg IV over 15–30 min	Once
Calcitonin	4–8 IU/kg SC	Q12–24 h
Gallium nitrate	200 mg/m^2 IV over 24 h	Qd x 5 d
Glucocorticoids	200–300 mg hydrocortisone IV	Qd x 5 d
Dialysis	—	—

Data from Bringhurst FR, Demay MB, Kronenberg HM. Hormones and disorders of mineral metabolism. In: Kronenberg HM, Melmed S, Polonsky KS, et al, editors. Williams textbook of endocrinology. 11th edition. Philadelphia: Saunders; 2008.

diuretic can be added to further augment urinary calcium excretion. Thiazide diuretics decrease urinary calcium excretion and should be avoided. Fluid status and electrolytes require strict monitoring to prevent overcorrection or fluid overload.[36]

Bisphosphonates have become the mainstay of treatment for hypercalcemia. They bind to bone hydroxyapatite and inhibit osteoclast formation and function, leading to decreased bone resorption. The most commonly used bisphosphonates in the United States, zoledronate and pamidronate, may be administered IV and are generally well tolerated. Studies of pamidronate report decreases in calcium levels in 24 hours, with normalization of calcium in 90% of patients in 3 to 4 days. These effects usually last for 3 to 4 weeks.[40] Pamidronate is much less expensive per dose; however, zoledronate has the advantage of ease of administration (see **Table 1**).

With the widespread use of bisphosphonates, the emergency physician should be aware of their potential toxicities. Up to one-third of patients report acute phase reactions usually within 2 days of treatment. The acute phase reactions, typically bone pain and flu-like symptoms, will resolve within 1 to 2 days. Patients are also at risk for hypophosphatemia, hypermagnesemia, and hypocalcemia. Close monitoring of electrolytes will allow for appropriate supplementation or treatment as indicated. The more feared complication of IV bisphosphonates is nephrotoxicity occurring in 6% to 10% of patients.[41] Patients with moderate renal insufficiency (glomerular filtration rate >30 mL/min) may still receive full dosing; however, it may be prudent to prolong the rate of delivery to 2 to 3 times the normal time of infusion. For more severe renal insufficiency, patient should forego bisphosphonates and instead undergo dialysis with low-calcium dialysate.[42] Recent literature also associates osteonecrosis of the jaw with bisphosphonate use. At particular risk are those patients with breast cancer or multiple myeloma with an incidence as high as 10%.[43] Ophthalmologic complications, such as anterior uveitis, scleritis, and conjunctivitis can also occur after administration.[41]

Other second-line agents may be of help when bisphosphonates fail or contraindications prevent their use. Salmon calcitonin increases renal excretion of calcium and decreased osteoclast-mediated bone resorption. Calcitonin has the most rapid reduction in calcium levels, with full results in 12 to 24 hours. However, the total reduction serum calcium is quite small and transient. Calcitonin has been shown to be more effective when combined with glucocorticoids. Steroids lower calcium levels by inhibiting the effects of vitamin D. They are particularly suited for treatment associated with lymphomas and elevated 1,25(OH)2 vitamin D. Steroids have a slow onset of action, and effects are not seen for 4 to 10 days.[36,44] Historically, plicamycin (mithramycin) was used to treat hypercalcemia before the wide availability of bisphosphonates. Although reported to be effective in up to 80% of patients, its use was limited by side effects that include renal insufficiency, hepatotoxicity, thrombocytopenia, and coagulopathy.[35] The manufacturer discontinued production in 2000 due to decreased demand. Gallium nitrate is also very effective in lowering calcium levels through potent inhibition of bone resorption. However, treatment requires a continuous infusion over 5 days and side effects, including pleural effusions, pulmonary infiltrates, optic neuritis, and nephrotoxicity, complicate its effectiveness.[45]

Occasionally, certain patients with severe hypercalcemia of malignancy may be poor candidates for standard therapy with IV fluids and bisphosphonates. In this situation, dialysis may be indicated. This would typically be reserved for patients with renal insufficiency or heart failure. The standard hemodialysis fluid must be modified to be virtually calcium-free. Other modifications to the dialysis fluid can be considered on an individual basis based on the particular electrolyte abnormalities of the patients.

For example, enrichment of the dialysate with phosphorus proved to result in rapid correction of all metabolic abnormalities after the patient had failed other medical therapy.

Disposition

Patients with severe hypercalcemia associated with malignancy will require close monitoring as treatment is begun to reduce calcium levels as well as diagnose and treat the underlying illness. An intensive-care setting may be required as the patient is initially rehydrated to watch for signs of electrolyte abnormalities with cardiac monitoring and frequent laboratory testing. These patients will need strict measurement of fluid input and output to determine overall hydration status. Ongoing care should be guided by response to treatment and overall underlying disease.

Future Directions

Although the majority of patients with hypercalcemia will respond to saline hydration and treatment with bisphosphonates, as many as one-quarter with HHM will fail to achieve normocalcemia. The resistance to treatment is attributed to renal calcium reabsorption and inadequate inhibition of bone resorption. New treatments are in development that target the molecular pathway leading to osteoclast recruitment and differentiation. This is known as the receptor activator of nuclear factor-kB (RANKL) ligand system. Monoclonal antibodies directed against RANKL and recombinant osteoprotegerin (OPG) are novel agents that interfere with this system. Animal studies comparing OPG to bisphosphonate to treat hypercalcemia of malignancy have been promising. Morony and colleagues reported rapid reversal of hypercalcemia with OPG, which occurred faster and lasted longer than treatments with bisphosphonates. Hypercalcemia eventually returned despite clear evidence of significantly suppressed bone resorption but to a lesser extent than those treated with bisphosphonates.[46] A small study in 2007 has also shown cinacalcet (calcimimetic) to be effective in lowering calcium levels in patients with elevated PTH related to parathyroid carcinoma. The patients had advance disease and had failed standard treatment with IV bisphosphonates and surgery. Two-thirds of the patients achieved a reduction in their serum calcium level of at least 1 mg/dL.[47]

These agents will require further testing to determine their overall safety and effectiveness in treating hypercalcemia of malignancy. It remains to be determined if they can be produced in a more cost effective manner as well as with better outcomes than those of standard treatment with bisphosphonates.

HYPOMAGNESEMIA

Hypomagnesemia frequently complicates the stay of hospitalized patients and seems to correlate with severity of illness. Up to 60% of patients in intensive care have low serum magnesium. Symptoms become present at levels below 1.2 mg/dL; however, they may be very nonspecific and are often overlooked. Most often, the symptoms manifest as neurologic or cardiovascular abnormalities. A neurologic examination may reveal muscle weakness, tremors, hyperreflexia, or tetany. Other neurologic abnormalities range from dizziness, apathy, and irritability to seizures and coma. Magnesium-deficient patients are also at risk for multiple dysrhythmias, ranging from atrial fibrillation, multifocal atrial tachycardia, and supraventricular tachycardia to premature ventricular contractions, ventricular tachycardia, or even ventricular fibrillation. Patients with congestive heart failure, who are treated with diuretics or digoxin, are particularly prone to dysrhythmias.[48]

Patients with any serious signs or symptoms of hypomagnesemia should be treated with IV magnesium. The standard dosage is 2 to 4 g of 50% magnesium sulfate diluted in saline or dextrose over 1 hour. Faster administration may result in bradycardia, heart block, or hypotension. These symptoms may be exacerbated with pre-existing renal insufficiency or atrioventricular block.

HYPOPHOSPHATEMIA

Hypophosphatemia is an additional electrolyte abnormality common to hospitalized patients. It is also a known complication of bisphosphonate treatment. Mild to moderate hypophosphatemia is usually asymptomatic; however, if the serum phosphate levels drop below 1.0 mg/dL, serious clinical symptoms may be present. The symptoms are related to impaired energy metabolism from decreased ATP production. As a result, all organ systems can be affected. Clinical signs and symptoms range from muscle weakness, rhabdomyolysis, impaired cardiac contractility, respiratory depression, confusion, seizures, and coma.

Although mild to moderate hypophosphatemia can be corrected with oral phosphate supplementation, severe symptomatic hypophosphatemia should be corrected with IV phosphate. Two standard formulations, potassium phosphate or sodium phosphate, are available for use in various suggested regimens. Weight-based regimens recommend 2.5 to 5 mg/kg over 6 hours.[49] More aggressive treatment with up to 30 mmol potassium phosphate IV in 50 mL saline over 2 h has also proven to be safe.[50] The faster replacement therapy takes place, the more likely that side effects will occur. Side effects of IV phosphate repletion include hypocalcemia, hyperkalemia, volume overload, hypernatremia, metabolic acidosis, and hyperphosphatemia.[51]

SUMMARY

A thorough working knowledge of the diagnosis and treatment of life-threatening electrolyte abnormalities in cancer patients, especially hyponatremia, hypoglycemia, and hypercalcemia, is essential to the successful practice of emergency medicine. Newer therapies that are targeted at the pathophysiological mechanisms underlying these electrolyte abnormalities have recently been developed and appear to have a promising future.

REFERENCES

1. Lee CT, Guo HR, Chen JB. Hyponatremia in the emergency department. Am J Emerg Med 2000;18:264–8.
2. Sverha JJ, Borenstein M. Emergency complications of malignancy. In: Tintinalli J, Kelen GD, Stapcyzinski JS, editors. Emergency medicine: a comprehensive study guide. 5th edition. New York: McGraw-Hill; 2000. p. 1408–14.
3. Cao L, Prashant J, Sumoza D. Renal salt wasting in a patient with cisplatin-induced hyponatremia. Am J Clin Oncol 2002;25:344–6.
4. Sorensen JB, Andersen MK, Hansen HH. Syndrome of inappropriate secretion of antidiuretic hormone (SIADH) in malignant disease. J Intern Med 1995;238: 97–110.
5. Johnson BE, Chute JP, Rushin J, et al. A prospective study of patients with lung cancer and hyponatremia of malignancy. Am J Respir Crit Care Med 1997;156: 1669–78.
6. Verbalis JG, Goldsmith SR, Greenberg A, et al. Hyponatremia treatment guidelines 2007: expert panel recommendations. Am J Med 2007;120:S1–21.

7. Yeong-Hau LH, Shapiro JI. Hyponatremia: clinical diagnosis and management. Am J Med 2007;120:653–8.
8. Vassal G, Rubie C, Kalifa C, et al. Hyponatremia and renal sodium wasting in patients receiving cisplatinum. Pediatr Hematol Oncol 1987;4:337–44.
9. Arieff A, Llach F, Massey SG. Neurological manifestations and morbidity of hyponatremia: correlation with brain water and electrolytes. Medicine 1976;55:121–9.
10. Lauriat SM, Berl T. The hyponatremic patient: practical focus on therapy. J Am Soc Nephrol 1997;8:1599–607.
11. Sterns RH. Severe symptomatic hyponatremia: treatment and outcome. A study of 64 cases. Ann Intern Med 1987;107:656–64.
12. Decaux G, Soupart A. Treatment of symptomatic hyponatremia. Am J Med Sci 2003;326(1):25–30.
13. Adams RD, Victor M, Mancall ED. Central pontine myelinolysis: a hitherto undescribed disease occurring in alcoholic and malnourished patients. AMA Arch Neurol Psychiatry 1959;81(2):154–72.
14. Wright DG, Laureno R, Victor M. Pontine and extrapontine myelinolysis. Brain 1979;102:361–5.
15. Rabinstein AA, Wijdicks EF. Hyponatremia in critically ill neurological patients. Neurologist 2003;9(6):290–300.
16. Yancey PH, Clark ME, Hand SC, et al. Living with water stress: evolution of osmolyte systems. Science 1982;217:1214–22.
17. Lien YH. Role of organic osmolytes in myelinolysis. A topographic study in rats after rapid correction of hyponatremia. J Clin Invest 1995;95:1579–86.
18. Soupart A, Decaux G. Therapeutic recommendations for management of severe hyponatremia: current concepts on pathogenesis and prevention of neurologic complications. Clin Nephrol 1996;46:149–69.
19. Laureno R. Central pontine myelinolysis following rapid correction of hyponatremia. Ann Neurol 1983;13:232–42.
20. Soupart A, Ngassa M, Decaux G. Therapeutic relowering of the serum sodium in a patient after excessive correction of hyponatremia. Clin Nephrol 1999;51:383–6.
21. Knepper MA. Molecular physiology of urinary concentrating mechanism: regulation of aquaporin water channels by vasopressin. Am J Phys 1997;272:F3–12.
22. Verbalis JG, Bisaha JG, Smith N. Novel vasopressin V1A and V2 antagonist (conivaptan) increases serum sodium concentration and effective water clearance in patients with hyponatremia. J Card Fail 2004;10(Suppl 4):S27.
23. Ghali JK, Koren MJ, Taylor JR, et al. Efficacy and safety of oral conivaptan: a V1A/V2 vasopressin receptor antagonist, assessed in a randomized, placebo-controlled trial in patients with euvolemic or hypervolemic hyponatremia. J Clin Endocrinol Metab 2006;91(6):2145–52.
24. Vaprisol (package insert). Deerfield (IL): Astellas Pharma US; 2005.
25. Oh M. Management of hyponatremia and clinical use of vasopressin antagonists. Am J Med Sci 2007;332:101–5.
26. Nayar MK, Lombard MG, Furlong NJ, et al. Diagnosis and management of non-islet cell tumor hypoglycemia. Endocrinologist 2006;16(4):227–30.
27. Service FJ. Hypoglycemic disorders. N Engl J Med 1995;91:505–10.
28. de Groot JW, Rikhof B, van Doorn J, et al. Non-islet cell tumour induced hypoglycaemia: a review of the literature including two new cases. Endocr Relat Cancer 2007;14:979–93.
29. Le Roith D. Tumor-induced hypoglycemia. N Engl J Med 1999;341:757–8.
30. Marks V, Teale JD. Tumours producing hypoglycaemia. Endocr Relat Cancer 1998;5:111–29.

31. Daughaday WH, Trivedi B. Measurement of derivatives of proinsulin-like growth factor-II in serum by radioimmunoassay directed against the E-domain in normal subjects and patients with nonislet cell tumor hypoglycemia. J Clin Endocrinol Metab 1992;75:110–5.
32. Strewler GJ. Humoral manifestations of malignancy. In: Kronenberg HM, Shlomo M, Polonsky KS, et al, editors. Williams textbook of endocrinology. 11th edition. Philadelphia: Saunders; 2008. p. 1803–17.
33. Mundy GR, Guise TA. Hypercalcemia of malignancy. Am J Med 1997;103: 134–45.
34. Ralston SH, Gallagher SJ, Patel U, et al. Cancer associated hypercalcemia: morbidity and mortality: clinical experience in 126 treated patients. Ann Intern Med 1990;112:499–504.
35. Barri YM, Knochei JP. Hypercalcemia and electrolyte disturbances in malignancy. Hematol Oncol Clin North Am 1996;10:775–80.
36. Stewart AF. Clinical practice. Hypercalcemia associated with cancer. N Engl J Med 2005;352(4):373–9.
37. Nussbaum SR, Gaz RD, Arnold A. Hypercalcemia and ectopic secretion of parathyroid hormone by an ovarian carcinoma with rearrangement of the gene for parathyroid hormone. N Engl J Med 1990;323:1324–8.
38. Ladenson JH, Lewis JW, McDonald JM, et al. Relationship of free and total calcium in hypercalcemic conditions. J Clin Endocrinol Metab 1978;48:393–7.
39. Shepard MM, Smith JW. Hypercalcemia. Am J Med Sci 2007;334(5):381–5.
40. Body JJ. Current and future directions in medical therapy: hypercalcemia. Cancer 2000;88:3054–8.
41. Layman R, Olson K, Van Poznak C. Bisphosphonates for breast cancer. Hematol Oncol Clin North Am 2007;21(2):341–67.
42. Koo WS, Jeon DS, Ahn SJ, et al. Calcium-free hemodialysis for the management of hypercalcemia. Nephron 1996;72:424–8.
43. Woo SB, Hellstein JW, Kalmar JR. Systematic review: bisphosphonates and osteonecrosis of the jaws. Ann Intern Med 2006;144(10):753–61.
44. Ariyan CE, Sosa JA. Assessment and management of patients with abnormal calcium. Crit Care Med 2004;32:S146–54.
45. Kinirons MT. Newer agents for the treatment of malignant hypercalcemia. Am J Med Sci 1993;305:403–6.
46. Morony S, Warmington K, Adamu S, et al. The inhibition of RANKL causes greater suppression of bone resorption and hypercalcemia compared with bisphosphonates in two models of humoral hypercalcemia of malignancy. Endocrinology 2005;146:3235–43.
47. Shoback D. Cinacalcet hydrochloride reduces hypercalcemia in patients with parathyroid carcinoma. Nat Clin Pract Endocrinol Metab 2007;3(12):794.
48. Gibbs MA, Tayal VS. Electrolyte disturbances. In: Marx JA, Hockberger RS, Walls RM, et al, editors. Rosen's emergency medicine: concepts and clinical practice. 6th edition. Philadelphia: Saunders; 2006. p. 1933–53.
49. Taylor BE, Huey WY, Buchman TG, et al. Treatment of hypophosphatemia using a protocol based on patient weight and serum phosphorus level in a surgical intensive care unit. J Am Coll Surg 2004;198(2):198–204.
50. Charron T, Bernard F, Skrobik Y. Intravenous phosphate in the intensive care unit: more aggressive repletion regimens for moderate and severe hypophosphatemia. Intensive Care Med 2003;29(8):1273–8.
51. Gaasbeek A. Hypophosphatemia: an update on its etiology and treatment. Am J Med 2005;118(10):1094–101.

Renal Complications in Oncologic Patients

Melissa L. Givens, MD, MPH[a,b,*], Joy Crandall, DO, FACMT[a]

KEYWORDS

- Acute renal failure • Tumor lysis syndrome
- Thrombotic microangiopathy • Nephrotoxicity • Malignancy

Acute renal failure (ARF) can be one of the many complications associated with malignancy and, unfortunately, often harbors a worse prognosis for the afflicted patient. Insult to the kidneys can occur for a variety of reasons in the oncologic patient. The kidneys are susceptible to injury from malignant infiltration, damage by metabolites of malignant cells, nephrotoxic drugs including chemotherapeutic agents, tumor lysis syndrome (TLS), radiation, septicemia associated with immune suppression, cast nephropathy, complications of bone marrow transplant (BMT), and autoimmune phenomena. This article focuses on several of these etiologies, such as TLS and thrombotic microangiopathy (TMA), which are unique threats faced by the oncologic patient. Therapeutic and diagnostic drug-induced nephrotoxicity, although common in all disease states, is also briefly reviewed. Nephrotoxic complications of chemotherapeutic agents warrant a separate discussion and are reviewed elsewhere in this issue.

EPIDEMIOLOGY

It is difficult to quantify the extent of renal complications associated with malignancy, as renal dysfunction can be present before the identification of malignancy, coincide with the diagnosis of malignancy, or be a secondary or tertiary effect of treatment. Several studies have examined the occurrence of renal failure in patients with specific malignancies, such as leukemia, lymphoma, and multiple myeloma. About 20% to 40% of newly diagnosed multiple myeloma patients have evidence of renal impairment.[1,2] Renal failure in lymphoma and leukemia is also well described. The incidence of renal complications in leukemia patients undergoing chemotherapy has been reported to be 30% or greater.[3,4] Patients undergoing BMT for leukemia have

A version of this article was previously published in the *Emergency Medicine Clinics of North America*, 27:2.

[a] Department of Emergency Medicine, Carl R. Darnall Army Medical Center, 36000 Darnall Loop, Fort Hood, TX 76544, USA

[b] Department of Military and Emergency Medicine, Uniformed Services University of the Health Sciences, 4301 Jones Bridge Road, Bethesda, MD, USA

* Corresponding author. Department of Emergency Medicine, Carl R. Darnall Army Medical Center, 36000 Darnall Loop, Fort Hood, TX 76544.

E-mail address: melissa.givens@us.army.mil

a 50% risk of renal complications.[4] Unfortunately, the presence of ARF is also an independent risk factor for a poor prognosis.[5–8] A reasonable approach to these patients in the emergency department (ED) is to consider prerenal, renal, and postrenal etiologies, since more than 1 type of azotemia may be present (listed in **Table 1**).[9]

PRERENAL AZOTEMIA

Prerenal azotemia is commonly encountered in cancer patients and can be due to multiple mechanisms, including poor oral intake, early satiety, vomiting, and diarrhea. Elderly cancer patients are particularly prone to dehydration, which should be corrected promptly to minimize further renal injury.

RENAL AZOTEMIA
Malignant Infiltration

Malignant infiltration of the kidneys is very common in leukemia and lymphoma. Fortunately, the presence of malignancy-related infiltration does not always coincide with renal dysfunction, and severe infiltration is rare.[10,11] Leukemic or lymphoma infiltration of the kidneys can present with a variety of signs and symptoms, varying from mild proteinuria to florid ARF. The only way to diagnose infiltration is by renal biopsy; thus, in the emergent evaluation of malignancy-associated renal failure, it is important to exclude more easily identifiable causes for the dysfunction.[10,11] Once identified, infiltration of the kidney is addressed by aggressively treating the primary malignancy with chemotherapy.

Tumor Lysis Syndrome

TLS is a metabolic emergency secondary to the breakdown of a large tumor burden with release of intracellular contents into the extracellular space and systemic circulation. Factors that contribute to TLS are the type of malignancy, its responsiveness to chemotherapy, rapidity of cell turnover, and tumor burden. It is clinically defined by the triad of hyperuricemia, hyperphosphatemia, and hyperkalemia, whereas elevated serum lactate dehydrogenase (LDH) levels, hypocalcemia, and ARF are secondary findings. Although the potassium and phosphate are primarily derived from

Table 1
Causes of acute renal failure in cancer patients

Prerenal Failure	Renal (Intrinsic) Failure	Postrenal Failure
Volume loss	Acute tubular necrosis	Intrarenal obstruction
Poor intake	Shock	Urate crystals
Diarrhea	Nephrotoxic compounds	Light chain (myeloma)
Vomiting	Intravascular hemolysis	Extrarenal obstruction
Sepsis	Acute interstitial nephritis	Retroperitoneal fibrosis
Drugs	Cancer infiltration	Ureteral/bladder outlet
NSAIDs	Postinfectious	obstruction
ACE inhibitors	glomerulonephritis	
Sinusoidal obstruction	Allergic nephritis	
syndrome (hepatorenal	Vascular nephritis	
syndrome)	Thrombotic	
Capillary leak syndrome (IL-2)	microangiopathy	
	Renal vasculature	
	thrombosis or stenosis	
	Glomerulonephritis	

Abbreviations: ACE, angiotensin-converting enzyme; IL-2, interleukin-2.

cytoplasmic contents, the uric acid is a product of nucleic acid breakdown. Hypocalcemia is secondary to calcium downregulation in the setting of hyperphosphatemia. TLS can occur spontaneously, but it is more commonly seen following the initiation of chemotherapy. Cancers such as acute lymphocytic leukemia (ALL), acute myelogenous leukemia (AML), Burkitt's lymphoma, and large solid tumors are more prone to TLS after the initiation of chemotherapy. Spontaneous TLS has been described in AML and ALL and is usually associated with marked hyperuricemia in the absence of hyperphosphatemia. It is thought that in spontaneous TLS, the released phosphorus is reutilized by new cancer cells.

TLS usually appears within 1 to 5 days of a chemotherapy session. Symptoms are nonspecific and include nausea, vomiting, fatigue, and weakness. Altered mental status, cardiac dysrhythmias, autonomic instability, and ARF are common findings on presentation. A recent study by Montesinos and colleagues[12] evaluated predisposing factors in an attempt to develop a predictive model for TLS in patients with AML. In this study of 772 adults, 130 (17%) developed TLS. Multivariate analysis showed that pretreatment LDH levels above laboratory normal values, creatinine (Cr) >1.4 mg/dL, uric acid >7.5 mg/dL, and white blood cell counts >25 × 10(9)/L were independent risk factors for TLS. Prechemotherapy laboratory evaluation should be performed to assess the risk for development of TLS and to assist in the decision to initiate prophylactic therapy in high-risk patients.

The goal of therapy and prophylaxis (**Table 2**) is to promote excretion of metabolic products, to prevent renal failure, and decrease uric acid production. The mainstay of therapy to date has been hydration or hyperhydration. Two to 4 times maintenance hydration with normal saline or isotonic sodium bicarbonate solutions to assist with urine alkalinization is generally recommended. Urine alkalinization with sodium bicarbonate to a goal pH between 7.0 and 8.0 may prevent precipitation of uric acid in the renal tubules; however, there are no experimental studies confirming any benefit to urine alkalinization. One study that compared urine alkalinization to hydration alone showed hydration to be just as effective in minimizing uric acid precipitation.[13] Furthermore, alkalinization may encourage deposition of calcium phosphate in organs of patients with existing hyperphosphatemia. Current recommendations are to alkalinize urine with a bicarbonate solution only in patients with existing metabolic acidosis. Alkalinization should continue until uric acid ceases to climb and is closer to a normal reference range of 2.0 to 8.0; however, reference ranges differ for males, females, and pediatric versus adult populations. If bicarbonate alkalinization fails to achieve a urine pH greater than 7.0, intravenous (IV) acetazolamide may be given to well-hydrated patients to decrease bicarbonate reabsorption in the proximal renal tubules.[14] Bicarbonate therapy should be discontinued once uric acid levels normalize, if serum bicarbonate is greater than 30 mEq/L, or if urine pH is more than 8.0. It is also important to simultaneously manage other symptomatic electrolyte abnormalities, such as hyperkalemia and hypocalcemia.

Allopurinol, rasburicase, and dialysis for renal failure are also appropriate adjunctive therapies to hydration. Allopurinol works by inhibiting xanthine oxidase, which prevents further production of uric acid but does nothing to decrease existing pools. Allopurinol also leads to increased levels of hypoxanthine and xanthine in the urine. Even when combined with hydration, allopurinol may fail to prevent renal compromise in up to 25% of cases.[15] Concurrent urine alkalinization with the use of allopurinol has been standard, but is now somewhat controversial. Rasburicase is a newer and highly effective alternative to allopurinol, which does not require simultaneous urine alkalinization. Rasburicase is a highly soluble IV recombinant form of urate oxidase, which can also be used to prevent or treat hyperuricemia. It acts by catalyzing the oxidation

Table 2
Tumor lysis syndrome drug therapies

Drug	Dosing	Mechanism
Acetazolamide	Oral: 5 mg/kg/dose repeated 2-3 times during 24 h	Inhibits carbonic anhydrase, increased renal excretion of sodium, potassium, bicarbonate, and water. Urine alkalization decreases urate crystal precipitation.
Allopurinol	Oral: 600-800 mg/d in 2-3 divided doses IV: 200–400 mg/m^2/d (max 600 mg/d)	Xanthine analog; competitively inhibits xanthine oxidase, blocks the metabolism of hypoxanthine and xanthine to uric acid. Decreases the formation of new uric acid. Reduce dosage by 50% in the setting of renal insufficiency.
Rasburicase	Low-risk with baseline uric acid <7.5 mg/dL—rasburicase 0.10 mg/kg Intermediate risk with baseline uric acid ≤7.5 mg/dL—rasburicase 0.15 mg/kg High-risk baseline uric acid level >7.5 mg/dL (450 mmol/L)—rasburicase 0.2 mg/kg	Catalyzes oxidation of uric acid to allantoin, which is more water soluble than uric acid and easily excreted.
Aluminum hydroxide	50–150 mg/kg/d divided every 4–6 h	Binds phosphate and bile salts to form an insoluble compound. Reduces serum phosphate levels. Risk of aluminum toxicity limits its use in renal failure.
Mannitol	0.5–1 g IV bolus	Increases the osmotic pressure of glomerular filtrate, preventing reabsorption of water and electrolytes and increasing urinary output. Increases phosphate excretion.

of uric acid to allantoin, which is 5 to 10 times more soluble in urine than in uric acid. Rasburicase effectively decreases levels of uric acid, xanthine, and hypoxanthine by reducing existing pools and preventing further production of uric acid. Although simultaneous hyperhydration is recommended, rasburicase does not require concomitant urine alkalinization and, thereby, also encourages phosphate excretion.[14] Several studies have verified its safety in pediatric as well as adult patients.[16] It is contraindicated in the setting of glucose-6-phosphate dehydrogenase deficiency, pregnancy, methemoglobinemia, or previous allergy and has a known side effect of hemolytic anemia. The 2008 International Expert Panel on TLS has provided rasburicase dosing guidelines based on the level of risk for TLS and uric acid levels, which can be found in **Table 2**.[17] Several small studies demonstrated effective treatment and prophylaxis for TLS and noted a decreased incidence of renal failure with the use of rasburicase.[18] One study of 11 patients showed a drop in uric acid to normal levels with a single dose regimen.[19,20] Rasburicase has shown promising results for treatment and prophylaxis of TLS as well as prevention of TLS-induced renal failure, though more large-scale studies are needed.

Hyperphosphatemia may be treated with oral phosphate binders, such as aluminum hydroxide, with careful observation for aluminum toxicity in the renally impaired patient. Mannitol should be given only for hyperphosphatemia refractory to aluminum hydroxide in a well-hydrated patient.[21] Dialysis should be considered early, especially in the presence of hyperphosphatemia greater than 10 mg/dL, ARF, extreme potassium abnormalities, or a calcium-phosphate product greater than 50. The calcium-phosphate product can be easily calculated by multiplying the serum phosphate and total serum calcium levels. A level greater than 50 promotes calcium-phosphate deposition in renal tubules and will exacerbate underlying renal insufficiency.

TLS is a true oncologic emergency that is both preventable and amenable to treatment. Consultation with the patient's oncologist and admitting service is necessary to support the patient's ability to successfully complete chemotherapy and prevent the complications of TLS.

Nephrotoxic Drugs

Although aggressive treatment of malignancy is the cornerstone of successful outcomes, the available therapies carry their own risk profile. Many of the agents commonly used in the treatment of patients with malignancy, unfortunately, are known to carry a risk of nephrotoxicity. Chemotherapeutic agents are well known for their myriad side effects, and the agents most notable for causing renal dysfunction include mitomycin, gemcitabine, platinum compounds, methotrexate, and ifosfamide. Non-chemotherapeutic drugs commonly used in the treatment of patients with malignancy that are well known threats to renal function include cyclosporine, tacrolimus amino-glycosides, and amphotericin B.

Cyclosporine

Cyclosporine is the mainstay of treatment in BMT patients to prevent graft versus host disease. Cyclosporine is a well-known nephrotoxin whose acute toxicity is related to renal vasoconstriction, leading to decreased renal blood flow and reduced glomerular filtration. Long-term sequelae include interstitial fibrosis and arteriopathy. Correlation of serum levels to renal impairment is the rationale behind careful monitoring. In fact, studies have shown that in a well-monitored setting, cyclosporine is not a contributor to dialysis-dependent renal failure in BMT patients.[22–24] In the compromised patient, treatment includes discontinuation of the drug. Low-dose dopamine infusion (2 mcg/kg/min) has been reported to reverse renal dysfunction.[25]

Tacrolimus

Tacrolimus is another immunosuppressive used for prophylaxis of transplant rejection and for graft versus host disease. Nephrotoxicity is a known complication, and in a study of patients receiving stem cell transplants, more than half the patients doubled their Cr. Hemolytic uremic syndrome has also been described with tacrolimus use.[26]

Aminoglycosides

Gentamicin and other aminoglycosides are antibiotics commonly used in the treatment of life-threatening infections often encountered in the oncologic patient. Amino-glycosides are nephrotoxins associated with renal tubular damage manifested by proteinuria, oliguria, and azotemia. Careful serum level monitoring is tantamount, since levels more than the therapeutic range correlate with renal insufficiency. Particular drug combinations, such as gentamicin-cephalothin, that are well known to act synergistically in precipitating renal compromise should be avoided.[6]

Amphotericin B

Use of Amphotericin B is reserved for life-threatening fungal infections due to the high incidence of nephrotoxicity. Mechanisms of injury include renal vasoconstriction and direct tubular injury. Renal injury from Amphotericin B is dose related and cumulative. Fortunately, renal impairment is usually reversible with cessation of the drug.

Contrast Agents

Contrast agent nephropathy is one of the most common causes of renal failure in the cancer patient and one of the most avoidable. Typically, contrast agent-induced nephropathy is reversible and resolves within a few weeks without dialysis. Unfortunately, in cancer patients, particularly those with multiple myeloma, the damage can be irreversible and lead to chronic dialysis. As with all patients, vigilance before contrast infusion can prevent most renal compromise. Correction of pre-existing hypovolemia, pre- and postcontrast infusion hydration, and judicious dosing of contrast agent are all successful strategies to prevent nephropathy. For high-risk patients, such as those with multiple myeloma, consideration should be given for the use of nonionic, iso-osmolar contrast agents as well as a lower dose. Consultation with a radiologist can facilitate a cost-effective strategy to reserve the use for high-risk patients susceptible to injury. Protective use of N-acetyl cysteine may be considered, although solid evidence of benefit is yet to be established.[27] In the ED, the risk of IV contrast dye may be outweighed by the need to perform the appropriate radiographic study to diagnose life-threatening conditions.

Complications of Bone Marrow Transplant

In addition to immunosuppression with nephrotoxic drugs, BMT carries its own risk of renal complications. In the early phase following BMT, microangiopathy and graft versus host disease are etiologic causes for renal dysfunction along with drug toxicity, with a higher incidence in allogenic transplants. The most common time frame for the development of ARF following BMT is during the first 3 weeks. A unique hepatorenal-like syndrome has also been described and may be seen in up to 90% of post-BMT patients with ARF.[22] This syndrome, which is due to damage within the hepatic sinusoids, presents with jaundice and portal hypertension preceding the ARF, sodium retention with associated edema, a high blood urea nitrogen (BUN)/Cr ratio, mild hyponatremia, and hypotension.

Approximately 6 weeks post-BMT, TMA, which resembles the hemolytic-uremic syndrome, may also occur. This syndrome of nephritis, severe hypertension with associated neurologic complications, microangiopathic anemia and thrombocytopenia, and renal failure occur in 15% to 20% of patients. Although there are many possible causes for TMA, total-body irradiation appears to be the major culprit.[22] Patients undergoing allogenic transplants who receive higher doses of whole-body irradiation have a higher rate of renal dysfunction (up to 45%). Supportive therapy is the mainstay of care in these patients. Late renal complications occurring after 100 days or more post-BMT are most commonly drug related.[4]

POSTRENAL AZOTEMIA
ExtraRenal Obstruction

ARF secondary to obstruction is a less common etiology for renal compromise but often amenable to treatment. Obstruction may be due to cancers of the kidney, bladder, or prostate or due to abdominal metastasis. Although hydronephrosis is a common finding, it may be absent early in the course of obstruction or when obstruction is partial. Diagnosis is made by abdominal imaging, most commonly renal ultrasonography. Relief of obstruction can be provided with a ureteral stent or percutaneous nephrostomy. Recovery of renal function is dependent on the time course and severity of obstruction.[9]

IntraRenal Obstruction

The hallmark of intra-renal obstructive etiologies is cast nephropathy, which occurs in patients with multiple myeloma. ARF is a common presenting diagnosis in patients with multiple myeloma and may be caused by amyloidosis and glomerular infiltration with light chains in addition to cast nephropathy. Cast nephropathy can be precipitated by hypovolemia, sepsis, urinary pH more than 7, or hypercalciuria. Therapy involves hydration, elimination of nephrotoxic compounds, urine alkalinization in patient with Bence-Jones proteinuria, and correction of hypercalcemia. Other therapy includes alkylating agents with high-dose steroids.[8] Plasma exchange may have some theoretical benefit in clearing light chains, but no survival benefit or decrease in dialysis dependence has been demonstrated.[28]

MANAGEMENT

In the emergent treatment of the oncologic patient with renal dysfunction, it is important to help identify the underlying cause of renal dysfunction, as the treatment for the various insults is diverse. A detailed history outlining the course of the patient's disease, recent symptoms, concurrent illness, chemotherapeutic regimen, and other medication therapy is paramount in the care of these patients. An electrocardiogram can be used to quickly screen for the presence of hyperkalemia, and in the appropriate setting, a bedside ultrasound or bladder scan can identify acute urinary retention. Laboratory markers including BUN, Cr, serum electrolytes, magnesium, phosphate, calcium, and uric acid levels as well as a urinalysis are essential in the evaluation of the oncologic patient with renal dysfunction. It is also important to include appropriate drug levels if indicated for nephrotoxic drugs, such as cyclosporine, tacrolimus, and aminoglycosides. Studies with nephrotoxic contrast medium should be avoided in the presence of renal dysfunction. Consultation with oncology and nephrology should be sought, as the management of these patients can be very complex. The recognition of the etiology for renal dysfunction along with appropriate aggressive treatment can influence the prognosis for survivorship in the patient with malignancy.

Studies describe a survival rate of 35% to 65% in leukemic patients with renal failure. The large amount of variability relates to the inclusion or exclusion of patients undergoing chemotherapy, BMT, and the presence or absence of multiorgan failure in studied groups.[4,7,29] Mortality is at least 30%, but mortality rates can be much higher in ARF patients admitted to the intensive care unit. Factors associated with a poor prognosis are similar for all patients with renal failure and include advanced age, sepsis, need for mechanical ventilation, and other organ failure.[7] Mortality for ARF patients with these comorbidities approaches 100%.[30]

SUMMARY

ARF is associated with a poor prognosis in cancer patients. Prevention, proactive surveillance, and aggressive therapy are all effective strategies that can diminish its impact on the patient with malignancy. A multidisciplinary approach to care is essential to optimize outcomes.

REFERENCES

1. Alexanian R, Barlogie B, Dixon D. Renal failure in multiple myeloma. Arch Intern Med 1990;150:1693–5.
2. Blade J, Fernandez-Llama P, Bosch F, et al. Renal failure in multiple myeloma: presenting features and predictors of outcome in 94 patients from a single institution. Arch Intern Med 1998;158:1889–93.
3. Cordonnier C, Vernant JP, Brun B, et al. Acute promyelocyctic leukemia in 57 previously untreated patients. Cancer 1985;55:18–25.
4. Munker R, Hill U, Kolb H. Renal complications in acute leukemias. Haematologica 1998;83:416–21.
5. Augustson BM, Begum G, Dunn JA, et al. Early Mortality after diagnosis of multiple myeloma: analysis of patients entered onto the United Kingdom Medical Research Trials between 1980–2002. Medical Research Council Working Party. J Clin Oncol 2005;23(36):9219–26.
6. Eckman LN, Lynch EC. Acute renal failure in patients with acute leukemia. South Med J 1978;71(4):382–5.
7. Harris KPG, Hattersley JM, Feehally J, et al. Acute renal failure associated with hematologic malignancies: a review of 10 years experience. Eur J Haematol 1991;47:119–22.
8. Kastritis E, Anagnostopoulos A, Roussou M, et al. Reversibility of renal failure in newly diagnosed multiple myeloma patients treated with high dose dexamethasone containing regimes and the impact of novel agents. Haematologica 2007; 92:546–9.
9. Darmon M, Ciroldi M, Thiery G, et al. Clinical Review: Specific aspects of acute renal failure in cancer patients. Crit Care 2006;10:211. Available at: http://ccforum.com/content/10/2/211. Accessed September 15, 2008.
10. Da'as N, Polliack A, Cohen Y, et al. Kidney involvement and renal manifestations in non-Hodgkin's lymphoma and lymphocytic leukemia: a retrospective study in 700 patients. Eur J Haematol 2001;67:158–64.
11. Rifkin SI. Acute renal failure secondary to chronic lymphocytic leukemia: a case report. Medscape J Med 2008;10(3):67.
12. Montesinos P, Lorenzo I, Martín G, et al. Tumor lysis syndrome in patients with acute myeloid leukemia: identification of risk factors and development of a predictive model. Haematologica 2008;93(1):67–74.
13. Conger JD, Falk SA. Intrarenal dynamics in the pathogenesis and prevention of acute urate nephropathy. J Clin Invest 1977;59(5):786–93.
14. Yamaguchi T, Sugimoto T, Imai Y, et al. Successful treatment of hyperphosphatemic tumoral calcinosis with long-term acetazolamide. Bone 1995;16(4): 247S–50S.
15. Coiffier B, Riouffol C. Management of tumor lysis syndrome in adults. Expert Rev Anticancer Ther 2007;7(2):233–9.
16. Goldman SC, Holcenberg JS, Finlestein JZ, et al. A randomized comparison between Rasburicase and allopurinol in children with lymphoma or leukemia at high risk for tumor lysis. Blood 2001;97(10):2998–3003.
17. Coiffier B, Altman A, Pui CH, et al. Guidelines for the management of pediatric and adult tumor lysis syndrome: an evidence-based review. J Clin Oncol 2008; 26:2767–78.
18. Pui CH, Mahmoud HH, Wiley JM, et al. Recombinant Urate oxidase for the prophylaxis or treatment of hyperuricemia in patients with leukemia or lymphoma. J Clin Oncol 2001;19(3):697–704.

19. McDonnell AM, Lenz KL, Frei-Lahr DA, et al. Single-dose rasburicase 6 mg in the management of tumor lysis syndrome in adults. Pharmacotherapy 2006;26(6): 806–12.

20. Hummel M, Reiter S, Adam K, et al. Effective treatment and prophylaxis of hyper-uricemia and impaired renal function in tumor lysis syndrome with low doses of rasburicase. Eur J Haematol 2007;80(4):331–6.

21. Razis E, Arlin ZA, Ahmed T, et al. Incidence and treatment of tumor lysis syndrome in patients with acute leukemia. Acta Haematol 1994;91(4):171–4.

22. Zager RA. Acute renal failure in the setting of bone marrow transplantation. Kidney Int 1994;46:1443–58.

23. Zager RA, O'Quigley J, Zager BK, et al. Acute renal failure following bone marrow transplantation: a retrospective study of 272 patients. Am J Kidney Dis 1989;13: 210–6.

24. Mihatsch MJ, Ryffel B. Renal side effects of cyclosporine A with special reference to autoimmune disease. Br J Dermatol 1990;122(Suppl 36):101–15.

25. Conte G, Dal Canton A, Sabbatini M. Acute cyclosporine renal dysfunction reversed by dopamine infusion in healthy subjects. Kidney Int 1989;36:1086–92.

26. Woo M, Przepiorka D, Ippoliti C. Toxicities of tacrolimus and cyclosporin A after allogeneic blood stem cell transplantation. Bone Marrow Transplant 1997;20: 1095–8.

27. Hoffman U, Fischereder M, Kruger B, et al. The value of N acetyl cysteine in the prevention of radiocontrast agent-induced nephropathy seems questionable. J Am Soc Nephrol 2004;15:407–10.

28. Clark WF, Stewart AK, Rock GA, et al, for the Canadian Apheresis Group. Plasma exchange when myeloma presents as acute renal failure: a randomized, controlled trial. Ann Intern Med 2005;143:774–84.

29. Lanore JJ, Brunet F, Pochard F, et al. Hemodialysis for acute renal failure in patients with hematologic malignancies. Crit Care Med 1991;19(30):346–51.

30. Lameire NH, Flombaum CD, Moreau D, et al. Acute renal failure in cancer patients. Ann Med 2005;37:13–25.

Neutropenic Enterocolitis

Robert L. Cloutier, MD, FAAEM

KEYWORDS

- Neutropenia • Enterocolitis • Typhlitis • Fever
- Chemotherapy • Cancer

Neutropenic enterocolitis (NE) is a poorly understood disease, originally described as a complication of pediatric leukemia. NE typically presents with fever, abdominal pain, and abdominal distension. The integrity of the bowel wall is compromised either as a direct result of chemotherapy or as an indirect result of neutropenia, leaving the bowel vulnerable to bacterial invasion, necrosis, and perforation. Affected patients can progress rapidly to the sepsis syndrome along with multisystem organ failure, which made early cases of NE almost uniformly fatal. Outcomes have improved over time but depend heavily on a timely diagnosis and swift intervention. The diagnosis of NE is associated with a relatively high degree of morbidity and mortality. Reported mortality rates currently vary between 0.8% and 26%, but others still report rates between 50% and 100%.[1–3]

Emergency department (ED) physicians are the front line of treatment for many neutropenic patients. Recent advances in cancer treatment are exposing patients to more advanced chemotherapeutic regimens, resulting in more frequent periods of absolute immunocompromise and hence more potential ED visits.[4] This article discusses the clinical presentation of NE, effective diagnostic strategies weighing the relative utilities of ultrasonographic imaging versus computed tomography (CT), and treatment options examining surgical versus medical approaches.

BACKGROUND AND STATE OF THE EVIDENCE

Necrotizing enterocolitis has long been acknowledged in the pediatric literature but has been relatively rare in adult patients. Over time, the term *neutropenic enterocolitis* has evolved to better appreciate the role that neutropenia plays in the pathogenesis of this condition. Early reports date back to 1933, when Cooke observed submucosal hemorrhage and appendiceal perforation in leukemic children (cited in Cunningham and colleagues[1]). More contemporary reports date to 1962, with a case series by

A version of this article was previously published in the *Emergency Medicine Clinics of North America*, 27:3.

Department of Emergency Medicine, Doernbecher Children's Hospital, Oregon Health & Science University, 3181 Sam Jackson Park Road, Portland, OR 97239, USA

E-mail address: cloutier@ohsu.edu

doi:10.1016/j.hoc.2010.03.005
0889-8588/10/$ – see front matter © 2010 Elsevier Inc. All rights reserved.

hemonc.theclinics.com

Amromin and Salomon (cited in Cunningham and colleagues[1]). They reported a large series of 69 adults with NE and acute leukemia or lymphoma over a 5-year period. These patients, characteristically, developed necrotizing enteric lesions shortly after intensive chemotherapy. Development of these enteric lesions was generally independent of patient response to chemotherapy. Interestingly, most patients experienced excellent therapeutic responses to their chemotherapy before the onset of NE.[1] The patients almost uniformly experienced abdominal pain, distension, leukopenia, and intestinal necrosis with histologic evidence of bacterial invasion of the mucosa and submucosa of the bowel wall.[1,5] All patients in this series succumbed to their disease after the development of NE.[5] NE has also been termed ileocecal syndrome or typhlitis.

The literature discussing NE is varied and characterized by numerous case reports and case series, illustrating cases of NE across a spectrum of patients, both with and without cancer. There is, however, only a single analysis of the current state of evidence regarding NE by Gorschlüter and colleagues.[6] In that review, no clinical trials or case control studies were cited in the NE literature. Overall, prospective studies were rare and did not tend to reflect the highest levels of scientific evidence. There are many unanswered questions, and our understanding of the pathophysiology of NE is sparse at best. Official diagnostic criteria are also difficult to find, as are firm guidelines for treatment. Thus, the overall grade assigned to evidence in this article is low, given the virtual absence of any meaningful prospective research or clinical trials. In an editorial response by Sherwood L. Gorbach, summing up the state of our poor understanding of NE, he aptly describes the challenges of fully grasping NE thus: "the diversity of the pathology is matched by the difficulty in establishing the diagnosis on the basis of only clinical findings."[2] What can be said, however, is that any progress made to date, to improve outcomes in NE, has been the result of rapid identification and aggressive intervention, frequently by frontline providers such as ED physicians.

CLINICAL PRESENTATION AND RISK FACTORS

Neutropenic patients presenting for care in the ED, after the administration of chemotherapy, represent a particularly high-acuity patient population, requiring a thoughtful and thorough evaluation for all potential sources of infection. Patients are routinely evaluated for potential sources of infection by chest radiography, complete blood counts, blood cultures, and urine analysis. Neutropenic patients, presenting with either generalized or focal abdominal pain, along with fever, should uniformly be considered at risk for NE.

Several specific chemotherapeutic agents have been implicated in the development of NE. These include, among others, taxane-based therapies (ie, paclitaxel and docetaxel), gemcitabine, cytosine arabinoside, vincristine, doxorubicin, cyclophosphamide, 5-fluorouracil, leucovorin, and daunorubicin[3–5,7,8] (**Box 1**). The types of malignancies involved are also varied. Initial reports almost exclusively cited NE as a complication of pediatric leukemias. Although leukemias and many forms of lymphoma comprise a large number of the cases of NE, a wide variety of solid tumors, including breast, lung, colorectal, and ovarian cancer, have also been implicated.[3,4,7,8]

Although most patients present with NE after chemotherapeutic treatment for cancer, there are a small number of reported cases presenting in leukemic patients before the initiation of chemotherapy or as their presenting event leading to diagnosis.[9–11] There is also a case report of a trauma patient who developed NE after receiving antibiotics for osteomyelitis.[12] The underlying cause in this case was

---

Box 1
Chemotherapeutic agents implicated in neutropenic enterocolitis

Paclitaxel

Docetaxel

Gemcitabine

Cytosine

Arabinoside

Vincristine

Doxorubicin

Cyclophosphamide

5 -Fluorouracil

Leucovorin

Daunorubicin

---

attributed to reversible neutropenia caused by nafcillin, used as part of a prolonged (>10 days) home intravenous antibiotic treatment course. Other cases have been reported in the context of AIDS, aplastic anemia, cyclic neutropenia, and immune-suppression for bone marrow transplantation or renal transplantation.[12,13] Although the variety of patients at risk extends beyond the realm of oncologic patients, the unifying theme across all of these case reports is the existence of absolute neutropenia. The onset of symptoms seems to be closely related to the nadir in the patient's white blood cell count.[14] It is critical that the evaluating physician remain vigilant and consider NE in any neutropenic patient and not only in oncologic patients. Important nononcologic causes of NE are summarized in **Box 2**.

Presenting abdominal signs and symptoms for patients with NE can be varied and elusive. Although many will present with high-grade fevers, their neutropenic state may make it more difficult for them to accurately localize infection.[3,5,12-14] Many patients present with vague cramp-like abdominal pain, vomiting, and diarrhea.[3,5,14] Right lower quadrant pain may be part of the presentation, with or without rebound tenderness.[3,5] Abdominal distension and peritoneal signs may be the harbinger of intestinal perforation. The process seems to have a predilection for the terminal ileum and cecum (hence the name ileocecal syndrome or typhlitis). This is postulated to be because of the distensibility of the cecum and its limited blood supply.[3] Common presenting signs and symptoms are summarized in **Box 3**.

In the face of neutropenia and concurrent direct chemotherapeutic damage to the intestinal mucosa, there is an alteration of the gut lining making it more vulnerable

---

Box 2
Reported nononcologic causes of neutropenic enterocolitis

AIDS

Nafcillin in the treatment of osteomyelitis

Aplastic anemia

Cyclic neutropenia

Bone marrow suppression for bone marrow or renal transplantation

Box 3
Common signs and symptoms of neutropenic enterocolitis
Vague cramp-like abdominal pain
Localized right lower quadrant abdominal pain
Abdominal distension
Diarrhea
Rebound tenderness may or may not be present

to bacterial invasion. NE may mimic the presentation of appendicitis and a host of other diagnostic possibilities, including colonic pseudo-obstruction, inflammatory bowel disease, pseudomembranous colitis, infectious colitis, and diverticulitis.[3]

Compromise of the intestinal mucosa leaves it vulnerable to invasion by a host of pathogenic bacteria. The subsequent production of endotoxins leads to bacteremia, necrosis, and hemorrhage. Organisms isolated from surgical specimens have included gram-negative rods, gram-positive cocci, clostridial species, enterococci, cytomegalovirus, *Candida* species, and *Clostridium difficile*.[3] These organisms may present alone or in combination. There are no data describing the discrete microbiology of NE or the combinations of pathogens associated with the presentations of NE. Organisms associated with cases of NE will reflect local patterns noted among other neutropenic patients in a given locale.

Considerations in the pediatric population closely mirror those in the adult population. A recent study by McCarville and colleagues[15] attempting to characterize typhlitis in childhood cancer notes many of the same uncertainties of a largely clinical diagnosis based on a variable triad of fever, neutropenia, and abdominal pain. They did note that patients older than 16 years were at greater risk for typhlitis than younger patients.

THE ROLE OF DIAGNOSTIC IMAGING: CT AND ULTRASOUND

Means for definitively establishing a diagnosis of NE remain difficult. A high degree of clinical suspicion will ultimately need to be complemented with the appropriate use of diagnostic imaging. Plain radiographs have limited utility in the diagnosis of NE because of nonspecific findings. Under ideal circumstances, a paucity of air in the cecum and/or the right colon, accompanied by evidence of pneumatosis, will be present.

Ultrasound and CT are the present mainstays for the diagnosis of NE. Current evidence seems to support the use of CT if there is a need for clearer delineation among multiple disorders capable of causing differing degrees of bowel wall thickening (BWT).[14,16–18] In these studies, NE characteristics, such as BWT, nodularity, presence of pneumatosis, and degree of distension, were better appreciated on CT. Ultrasound may have advantages in terms of ascertaining the existence of BWT and rapidly ruling out other entities in the differential diagnosis, including appendicitis, intussusception, cholecystitis, or pancreatitis. The prognostic significance of BWT seen on ultrasound is a matter of some debate, with measurements exceeding 10 mm indicating a poor outcome.[5,14,16] There is a significant degree of overlap in measurements of BWT among neutropenic patients, limiting the diagnostic potential of ultrasonography in the ED.[7] This consideration becomes important in a patient with neutropenia and abdominal pain when there is a greater need to characterize the differences between NE, *C difficile* colitis and potential graft-versus-host disease (GVHD) in the bone marrow transplant patient. A study by Kirkpatrick and Greenberg retrospectively characterized the CT features of neutropenic patients with radiographic bowel abnormalities.[18] Their findings note numerous differences between the 3 entities described earlier, in terms of their CT appearance. NE was best characterized by its predilection for the right colon and cecum, with episodic appearances in the small bowel. It was also noted to exhibit the greatest degree of pneumatosis and mesenteric stranding as compared with GVHD or *C difficile* colitis.[18]

For the ED physician, the hemodynamic stability of the patient is of paramount importance in determining which imaging modality to use. Patients able to safely tolerate transport to the CT scanner will benefit from a more detailed imaging modality compared with ultrasound. CT may also help narrow the differential diagnosis by characterizing the extent and nature of the BWT (**Fig. 1**).

Patients who are hemodynamically unstable may benefit from the rapid detection of BWT using ultrasound, which can be performed at the bedside. For patients who are critically ill, the ED physician should request emergent surgical consultation for potential operative resection of necrotic bowel.

TREATMENT: MEDICAL VERSUS SURGICAL

Early case series of NE demonstrated a preference for surgical intervention.[5] Early and definitive resection of the ischemic bowel was associated with significant reductions in overall mortality from NE. Heterogeneity of the disease process and its myriad presentations, coupled with its incredibly high mortality rate, led many to believe in early surgical therapy for all patients with NE. As experience with the disease has increased, a greater proportion of the cases have been successfully managed medically, using aggressive hemodynamic support, bowel rest, and broad-spectrum antibiotic therapy with surgery reserved for the more severe cases.[5,6,14]

Antibiotic recommendations for patients with NE are numerous and varied. The Infectious Disease Society of America published a lengthy series of guidelines for antibiotic use in neutropenic patients with cancer in 2002.[19–23] Unfortunately, these guidelines only offer vague recommendations regarding abdominal infections. Overall, the

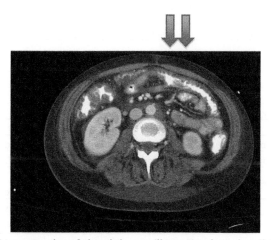

Fig. 1. Computed tomography of the abdomen illustrating bowel wall thickening associated with neutropenic enterocolitis. This is most notable in the upper portions of the image surrounded by intraluminal contrast (*arrows*).

choice of antibiotics should seek to cover a broad spectrum of gram-positive and gram-negative organisms as well as *Pseudomonas*, *C difficile*, and fungal organisms, such as *Candida* species. Monotherapies, such as piperacillin-tazobactam or imipenem-cilastatin, are good initial choices. Duotherapies, combining another beta-lactam antipseudomonal agent with an aminoglycoside or, alternatively, cefepime or ceftazidime coupled with metronidazole, are also acceptable. Anaerobic coverage is important primarily when using a cephalosporin monotherapy.[6] Recommended doses for adults and children are summarized in **Table 1**.

An interesting correlation between the recovery of the leukocyte count and improving clinical status has led to the notion of actively normalizing the leukocyte count by using the recombinant granulocyte colony stimulating factor (G-CSF) to hasten bowel healing.[3,6] Presently, there are no controlled trials governing the use of these agents.[6] Evidence to date suggests that they should be reserved for patients with the greatest degree of neutropenia (absolute neutrophil count <100/mL), severe uncontrolled disease, multisystem organ failure, and pneumonia accompanied by invasive fungal infection.[6]

In the case of a confirmed or high-likelihood diagnosis of NE, it is important for the ED physician to organize appropriate critical care resources and to obtain surgical consultation. Although several patients may recover with attentive and timely medical management, the potential for acute clinical decompensation, requiring operative intervention, must be anticipated. Primary treatment for a patient with NE is the same as that for other patients at risk for acute sepsis and hemodynamic collapse. An appropriate assessment of the ABCs should include adequate venous access for aggressive fluid support in addition to broad-spectrum antibiotics. Central venous access and an arterial line may be necessary if goal-directed therapy for sepsis is

Table 1
Antibiotics for empiric treatment of adult and pediatric neutropenic enterocolitis

Antibiotics for Empiric Treatment	Dosages
In adult neutropenic enterocolitis	
Monotherapy	
Piperacillin-tazobactam	3.375 g IV Q6 h
Imipenem-cilastatin	500 mg IV Q6 h or 1 g IV Q6–8 h
Duotherapy	
Ceftazidime	1 g IV Q8–12 h *or*
Cefepime	2 g IV Q8 h *plus*
Metronidazole	1 g IV Q6 h
In pediatric (1–12 y of age) neutropenic enterocolitis	
Monotherapy	
Piperacillin-tazobactam	(>9 mo and <40 kg) 300 mg/kg/d IV divided Q8 h.
Imipenem-cilastatin	(>3 mo) 60–100 mg/kg/d IV divided Q6 h, max: 2–4 g/d
Duotherapy	
Ceftazidime	90–150 mg/kg/d IV divided Q8 h max 6 g/d *or*
Cefepime	50 mg/kg IV Q8 h, max: 2 g/dose *plus*
Metronidazole	30 mg/kg/d IV divided Q6 h max 4 g/d

Abbreviations: IV, intravenous; Q, every.
Data from Gorschlüter M, Mey U, Strehl J, et al. Neutropenic enterocolitis in adults: systematic analysis of evidence quality. Eur J Haematol 2005;75:1–13.

desired. Lastly, a vigilant eye must be kept on any acute changes in the abdominal examination and the hemodynamic profile of the patient, pending transfer to an intensive care unit or operative setting.

SUMMARY

NE is a relatively rare but potentially devastating complication of neutropenic fever. Although it is poorly understood pathophysiologically, the importance of early diagnosis and intervention is clear. ED physicians, as frontline practitioners, have an important role in the continuum of care for many neutropenic patients. Patients presenting with fever, neutropenia (from any cause), and abdominal pain should all be considered at risk for NE. Early definitive imaging with CT, as a first choice in stable patients, should be performed in a timely manner. Treatment should include bowel rest, broad-spectrum antibiotics, and hemodynamic support if necessary. Early consultation with critical care specialists and surgery should be strongly considered.

REFERENCES

1. Cunningham SC, Fakery K, Bass BL, et al. Neutropenic enterocolitis in adults: case series and review of the literature. Dig Dis Sci 2005;50:215–20.
2. Gorbach SL. Neutropenic enterocolitis. Clin Infect Dis 1998;27:700–1.
3. Davila ML. Neutropenic enterocolitis. Curr Opin Gastroenterol 2006;22:44–7.
4. Kouroussis C, Samonis G, Androulakis N, et al. Successful conservative treatment of neutropenic enterocolitis complicating taxane-based chemotherapy: a report of five cases. Am J Clin Oncol 2000;23:309–13.
5. Wade DS, Nava HR, Douglas HO Jr. Neutropenic enterocolitis: clinical diagnosis and treatment. Cancer 1992;69:17–23.
6. Gorschlüter M, Mey U, Strehl J, et al. Neutropenic enterocolitis in adults: systematic analysis of evidence quality. Eur J Haematol 2005;75:1–13.
7. Geisler JP, Schraith DE, Manahan KJ, et al. Gemcitabine associated vasculitis leading to necrotizing enterocolitis and death in women undergoing primary treatment for epithelial ovarian/peritoneal cancer. Gynecol Oncol 2004;92:705–7.
8. Kronawitter U, Kemeny NE, Blumgart L. Neutropenic enterocolitis in a patient with colorectal carcinoma: unusual course after treatment with 5-fluorouracil and leucovorin—a case report. Cancer 1997;28:1–19.
9. Kaste SC, Flynn PM, Furman WL. Acute lymphoblastic leukemia presenting with typhlitis. Med Pediatr Oncol 1997;28:209–12.
10. Hsu T, Huang H, Yen D, et al. ED presentation of neutropenic enterocolitis in adult patients with leukemia. Am J Emerg Med 2004;22:276–9.
11. de Britto D, Barton E, Spearks KL, et al. Acute right lower quadrant pain in a patient with leukemia. Ann Emerg Med 1998;32:98–101.
12. Bibbo C, Barbieri RA, Deitch EA, et al. Neutropenic enterocolitis in a trauma patient during antibiotic therapy for osteomyelitis. J Trauma 2000;49:760–3.
13. Cutrona AF, Blinkhorn RJ, Crass J, et al. Probable neutropenic enterocolitis in patients with AIDS. Rev Infect Dis 1991;13:828–31.
14. Song HK, Krisel D, Canter R, et al. Changing presentation and management of neutropenic enterocolitis. Arch Surg 1998;133:979–82.
15. McCarville MB, Adelman CS, Chenghong L, et al. Typhlitis in childhood cancer. Cancer 2005;104:380–7.
16. Cartoni C, Dragoni F, Mixozzi A, et al. Neutropenic enterocolitis in patients with acute leukemia: prognostic significance of bowel wall thickening detected by ultrasonography. J Clin Oncol 2001;19:756–61.

17. Gorschluter M, Marklein G, Hofling K, et al. Abdominal infections in patients with acute leukemia: a prospective study applying ultrasonography and microbiology. Br J Haematol 2002;117:351–8.

18. Kirkpatrick ID, Greenberg HM. Gastrointestinal complications in the neutropenic patient: characterization and differentiation with abdominal CT. Radiology 2003; 226:668–74.

19. Teefey SA, Montana MA, Goldfogel GA, et al. Sonographic diagnosis of neutropenic typhlitis. AJR Am J Roentgenol 1987;149:731–3.

20. Hughes WT, Armstrong D, Bodey GP, et al. 2002 guidelines for the use of antimicrobial agents in neutropenic patients with cancer. Clin Infect Dis 2002;34: 730–51.

21. Williams N, Scott AD. Neutropenic colitis: a continuing surgical challenge. Br J Surg 1997;84:1200–5.

22. Katz JA, Wagner ML, Gresik MV, et al. Typhlitis. An 18-year experience and postmortem review. Cancer 1990;65:1041–7.

23. Shamberger RC, Weinstein HJ, Delorey MJ, et al. The medical and surgical management of typhlitis in children with acute nonlymphocytic (myelogenous) leukemia. Cancer 1986;57:603–9.

Myeloproliferative Disorders and the Hyperviscosity Syndrome

Bruce D. Adams, MD, COL, MC, US Army[a,b],*, Russell Baker, DO[c],
J. Abraham Lopez, MD[c], Susan Spencer, MD[c]

KEYWORDS

- Hyperviscosity syndrome • Essential thrombocytosis
- Hyperleukocytosis • Leukostasis • Polycythemia vera
- Waldenstrom macroglobulinemia

One of the most striking complications in hematologic disease is the development of acute blood hyperviscosity. Classically, hyperviscosity presents with the triad of bleeding, visual disturbances, and focal neurologic signs.[1] Hyperviscosity occurs from pathologic elevation of either the cellular or acellular (protein) fractions of the circulating blood.[2] In cellular fractions, significant elevation of any of the three primary blood cell lines may lead to clinical manifestations: erythrocytosis (red blood cells [RBC]), leukocytosis (white blood cells [WBC]) and thrombocytosis (platelets) (**Figs. 1** and **2**).[3] The term "hyperviscosity syndrome" (HVS) is best reserved for pathologic increases in circulating serum proteins, which also manifest with emergency signs and symptoms.[4] Although the underlying disease processes vary, general management measures for any of these conditions include aggressive supportive resuscitation, rapid reduction of the offending biologic substance, and definitive chemotherapeutic management of the underlying hematologic condition.[3,5] Emergency medicine providers should be aware of these conditions and be prepared to rapidly initiate supportive and early definitive management. This article is separated into four sections. The first section reviews classic HVS related to hyperproteinemia.

A version of this article was previously published in the *Emergency Medicine Clinics of North America*, 27:3.

[a] Department of Clinical Investigation, William Beaumont Army Medical Center, 5005 North Piedras Street, El Paso, TX 79920-5001, USA
[b] Department of Emergency Medicine, Medical College of Georgia, Augusta, GA, USA
[c] Department of Emergency Medicine, Texas Tech University Heath Sciences Center, Paul L. Foster School of Medicine, 4801 Alberta Avenue, El Paso, TX 79905, USA
* Corresponding author. Department of Clinical Investigation, William Beaumont Army Medical Center, 5005 North Piedras Street, El Paso, TX 79920-5001.
E-mail address: bruce.adams@amedd.army.mil

Hematol Oncol Clin N Am 24 (2010) 585–602
doi:10.1016/j.hoc.2010.03.004
0889-8588/10/$ – see front matter © 2010 Elsevier Inc. All rights reserved.

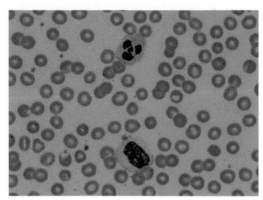

Fig. 1. A normal peripheral blood smear (hematoxylin-eosin, original magnification 1000x). (*Courtesy of* David Rankin, MD, El Paso, TX and Domingo Rosario, MD, El Paso, TX.)

The remainder of the article discusses the three basic lines of myeloproliferative disorders.

HVS RELATED TO HYPERPROTEINEMIA

Waldenstrom macroglobulinemia (WM) is the most common cause of HVS.[6] However, WM is a fairly rare disease with an incidence of only three per million persons annually (accounting for 1% to 2% of hematologic cancers).[6] The mean age at onset of WM is about 65 years with a slight predominance in men.[7] More than 30% all WM patients may develop HVS at some point.[8,9] Under the World Health Organization (WHO) classification scheme, WM is classified separately from the myelomas.[10]

Myelomas manifest HVS less frequently than WM but they are still the second leading cause of HVS. IgA myeloma is responsible for approximately 25% of cases

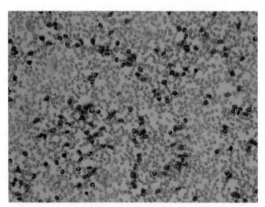

Fig. 2. Hyperleukocytosis in the setting of AML. This low power photomicrograph (hematoxylin-eosin, original magnification 10x) of a peripheral blood smear shows a markedly increased number of large (2–3 times the diameter of normal red blood cells). These cells display a high nuclear to cytoplasmic ratio. The total white blood cell count is well over 100,000/mm³ with about 60% to 70% blasts. Whereas blasts may be seen in regular bone marrow on up to 5% of the population, they are not a normal finding in peripheral blood. These large distended cells do not deform or easily traverse through the microcirculation causing hyperviscosity. (*Courtesy of* Thomas Repine, MD, El Paso, TX.)

of HVS followed by IgG myelomas at less than 5% of cases.[1] Light chain disease is also a commonly reported cause of HVS.[5] Polyclonal gammopathies from chronic infections or inflammatory disease may on occasion yield sufficiently high protein levels to create HVS, and usually respond to the same general treatment. Sjögren syndrome, rheumatoid arthritis, systemic lupus erythematosus, cryoglobinemia, diabetes mellitus, and even HIV, have been associated with HVS.[11-13]

Pathophysiology

Viscosity is formally defined as the internal frictional resistance of fluid to flow, or in simple terms, the "thickness" of the fluid.[14,15] Water has a lower viscosity than syrup; it therefore travels faster and easier, especially through small passageways.[15] Similarly, hyperviscous blood creates sludge and stasis in the capillary beds resulting in clinical manifestations at the tissue and circulatory level.[16] Viscosity derives from physical and chemical properties, most notably the concentration, the size, and the shape of the molecules. Centipoise (cp) is the standard unit for measuring dynamic fluid viscosity, named in honor of the French physiologist Jean Louis Marie Poiseuille (who also described Poiseuille's Law). Water has a viscosity of 1.00 cp at 20°C The large protein IgM pentameters in WM are highly viscous but HVS can also be seen in kappa light chain disease, which tends to form unstable, asymmetric, highly polymerized circulating aggregates.[4,5] The clinical manifestations of HVS appear when the serum viscosity relative to water is greater than about 3 cp; at higher levels of 4cp and 5cp the prevalence of HVS rises to 67% and 75%, respectively.[17] The underlying physiology of the patient creates significant variability from one patient to another, but for a given patient symptoms will manifest at about the same level of viscosity over time.[4]

Clinical Presentation

HVS should be considered in at least three different Emergency Department (ED) scenarios: the patient presenting with the classic triad of HVS; the ED patient who has a previously established immunoglobulin-producing hematologic diagnosis; and critically ill patients with certain laboratory clues pointing to a concurrent underlying gammopathy.

The classic presentation triad for HVS consists of bleeding, visual disturbances, and focal neurologic signs. However, a variety of end organ damage can be observed.[17] The bleeding typically arises from oozing mucosal surfaces including epistaxis, bleeding gums and gastrointestinal hemorrhage due to a supposed mechanism of impaired platelet function.[1,18] Retinopathy caused by thrombosis, microhemorrhage, exudates, and papilledema results in the common visual derangements.[19] These findings can be directly observed under fundoscopy with the classic picture of "sausage link" or "boxcar" venous engorgement of the retinal veins.[5] Neurologic complications may present with headache, generalized stupor, and coma, or focal findings including vertigo, hearing impairment, seizures, and stroke syndromes.[4,20,21] Not in the diagnostic triad, but often more hazardous, are the cardiopulmonary complications of HVS.[4,22] Among other mechanisms, the effectively expanded plasma volume seen in HVS may drive demand beyond cardiac reserve resulting in high output cardiac failure, valvular dysfunction, or myocardial infarction.[6]

Physicians should consider the diagnosis of HVS if a patient presents with unexplained neurologic symptoms such as visual change or headache in the setting of a concomitant immunoglobulin-producing hematologic condition.[21,23] HVS is often the presenting characteristic of dysproteinemias. Renal failure has been reported with HVS but is generally more common in myelomas. One mechanism of renal failure in HVS may be that the glomeruli are exposed to a relative hypoperfused "pre-renal" state.[24] Judicious hydration and avoiding use of diuretics is important to prevent further morbidity.[5,25] Myeloma patients are notoriously susceptible to radiologic contrast nephropathy, so great caution should be exercised in its administration. HVS is also one cause of symmetric peripheral gangrene of the extremities.[26]

Laboratory evaluation should include a complete blood cell count, full serum chemistries, and coagulation profiles.[1] Significant proteinuria on routine urinalysis and an elevated albumin-protein gap (albumin − protein difference) suggests an underlying gammopathy. Occasionally, the laboratory will report the presence of rouleaux formation on the peripheral blood smear or that they are unable to complete tests because the viscous serum has clogged their analytical instruments.[5,27] Paraneoplastic signs of multiple myeloma include hypercalcemia and hyponatremia.[2,22] Confirmatory serum and urine protein electrophoresis with the characteristic monoclonal spike on serum electrophoresis confirms an existing gammopathy; this test can be arranged in conjunction with the admitting physician.[28]

Diagnosis

HVS is a clinical diagnosis made on a combination of the symptoms discussed earlier in conjunction with a viscosity of 4 cp or greater as measured by a viscosimeter (normal viscosity is 1.4–1.8 cp).[28,29] Controversy exists on whether plasma viscosity or whole blood viscosity is better, but measurement of whole blood viscosity is probably superior to that of serum or plasma viscosity alone.[1,14] Laboratories report whole blood viscosity as comparable to a sample with a certain hematocrit (a viscosity comparable to that of a patient with a hematocrit of 70%). A relative whole blood viscosity of 55% or greater increases the risk of HVS.

Management

Physicians should base treatment decisions primarily on the severity of signs and symptoms rather than the measured degree of hyperviscosity.[1,5,8] HVS therapy can be viewed in 4 phases: supportive therapy, plasma exchange, plasmapheresis, and chemotherapy for the underlying hematologic condition. Specific chemotherapy is generally applied after the ED course by hematology/oncology consultants and is therefore beyond the scope of this article.[6,23]

Supportive Therapy

Paradoxically, these patients may be dehydrated yet present with high output cardiac failure. Judicious fluid resuscitation is usually necessary and diuretics should be avoided. Electrolyte derangements should be corrected with the foreknowledge that sodium derangements are often spurious. Antibiotics should be administered if any suspicion of infection exists. Although fluid compartment shifts may result in a measured anemia, these patients generally have a normal or supernormal red blood cell mass. Because packed red blood cell transfusions increase blood viscosity and thereby accelerate the HVS, they should be withheld until the viscosity can be measured and lowered appropriately.[1,17]

Plasma Exchange

In the ED, one temporizing measure in a patient with severe HVS is to perform an emergency plasma exchange. The procedure involves phlebotomizing between 1 and 2 units of blood from the patient while simultaneously replacing the volume with normal saline.[5,17] This therapy is of proven benefit and some experts believe it is more effective than plasmapheresis in decreasing serum viscosity in patients with

WM.[30,31] However, aggressive plasma exchange can deplete platelets, clotting factors, and albumin.[8,30] Emergency plasma exchange is indicated in the presence of severe neurologic findings (seizure or coma).[5] Measuring quantitative immunoglobulins before and after plasma exchange can help guide further hospital therapy but does not influence the ED course. IgA and IgG molecules have a higher volume of distribution (compared with the IgM of WM) and therefore plasma exchange may need to be performed more aggressively in these myelomas.[4,17]

Plasmapheresis

Plasmapheresis is the definitive treatment for HVS. The ED physician should establish large-bore central venous access while awaiting the plasmapheresis team, preferably with a dialysis catheter. As noted, IgG- or IgA-related HVS will require longer and more frequent plasmapheresis treatments. The IgM found in WM is mostly intravascular and therefore is cleared more readily. The major complication of plasmapheresis is hypocalcemia related to citrate binding from automated plasmapheresis systems.

ERYTHROCYTOSIS AND POLYCYTHEMIA VERA

Erythrocytosis results from an increase in the red cell mass with concomitant increase in RBC number, red cell count, and hematocrit.[32–34] This finding may be generally attributed to hemoconcentration given the many cases of dehydration, hypovolemia and other relative low-volume states encountered in the ED.[35] However, the critically ill patient presenting with an acute increase in hematocrit or in association with increases in other blood cell components (ie, platelets, leukocytes) requires consideration of a more aggressive diagnostic workup.[32]

The incidence of polycythemia vera (PCV) is about 2.6 cases per 100,000 persons, and is highest among Ashkenazi Jews.[36] PCV is associated with a point mutation of an autoinhibitory Janus kinase 2 (JAK2) protein kinase domain.[37,38] The activation of this domain results in erythropoeisis losing its dependence on erythropoietin signaling and becoming virtually autonomous.[39] Recent studies have identified several additional mutations within the JAK2 gene site that are now considered essential to the diagnosis of PCV.[32,38]

Pathophysiology

Hematopoiesis exists in a homeostatic balance between the body's requirements for particular blood cell lines and loss or destruction of those cells.[36] In the red cell line this balance is maintained by a feedback mechanism primarily involving the hormone erythropoietin.[36] Erythropoietin is primarily produced in the renal cortex, accounting for 90% of this circulating protein.[40] Secondary sites of production consist of liver, spleen, lung, testis, brain, and erythroprogenitor cells. Erythropoietin stimulation results in the production of 2×10^{11} red blood cells per day.[41] All blood cell lines arise from a common hematopoetic stem cell. These stem cells begin their initial differentiation onto erythrocyte progenitors when stimulated by one of several cytokine factors.[39,42]

Erythrocytosis is the proper term for a state of increase in circulating red cells. Specifically, PCV possesses these additional features and has potential for progression to advanced disease. Erythrocytosis is initially identified by the increased in hematocrit and red blood cell count, but it is important to remember that these indices are dependent on red blood cell mass and plasma volume.[43] Thus, a relative erythrocytosis occurs in cases of dehydration and low volume due to hemoconcentration. Correction in these cases can be accomplished by volume replacement and the condition may be short-lived.

An absolute erythrocytosis is associated with an increase in red cell production and mass. These patients are euvolemic with an increased hematocrit.[44] Absolute erythrocytosis has been classified as either primary or secondary.[45] Secondary erythrocytosis consists of congenital and acquired disorders. Congenital conditions are related to high oxygen affinity hemoglobinopathies and gene mutations (eg, 2,3-diphosphoglycerate deficiency).[46–48] Acquired conditions are associated with erythropoietin-mediated erythrocyte production. This erythropoietin response may be hypoxia in patients living in high altitudes, those with chronic lung disease, or from paraneoplastic effects.[39,49,50]

Diagnosis

The diagnosis begins with determining the red cell mass/body surface area in patients presenting with a persistently increased hematocrit in the absence of secondary causes of erythrocytosis. The Polycythemia Vera Study Group and the World Health Organization (WHO) have issued criteria for the diagnosis of PCV (**Box 1**).[51,52] New, proposed WHO criteria incorporate the presence of erythrocytosis or increased red cell mass and the presence of a known PCV molecular lesion.[51]

Treatment

Phlebotomy and low-dose aspirin are the mainstays of PCV treatment. The current recommendations are phlebotomy to a hematocrit of $\leq$45% in men and $\leq$42% in women.[36] However, no evidence exists for this goal of phlebotomy other than correlation between increased risk of thrombosis and a hematocrit >45% in these patients.[48] Low-dose aspirin (either 81 or 100 mg daily) is recommended unless there are specific contraindications.[36,53] More recent studies support initiation of aspirin therapy even in those patients with a previous history of gastric bleeding in the setting of concurrent use of a proton pump inhibitor.[43,54] Further treatment is individualized based on the patient's risk for thrombotic complications. A history of thrombosis, age more than 60 years, and associated thrombocytosis are indications for more aggressive treatment.[55]

The next step in the management of higher risk patients is the addition of cytoreductive therapy.[36,56] Options include hydroxyurea, chlorambucil, or intravenous radioactive phosphorus-32.[55] Recombinant interferon alpha is another option in

---

Box 1
Diagnosis of polycythemia vera (PCV) requires meeting either both major criteria and one minor criterion, or the first major criterion and two minor criteria

Major Criteria

Hemoglobin >18.5 g/dL in men

    Hemoglobin >16.5 g/dL in women

    Or increase red cell volume

    Presence of JAK2V617F or JAK2 exon 12 mutation

Minor Criteria

    PCV bone marrow changes

    Low serum erythropoietin level

    Endogenous erythroid colony formation in vitro

Data from Ref.[113]

myelosuppressive management.[55] Secondary erythrocytosis may be managed initially with phlebotomy. However, definitive management will require the primary cause to be addressed.[36] Malignancy, hypoxia, and extrinsic sources of erythropoietin should be addressed and managed accordingly. These patients are also at risk for neurologic sequelae.

HYPERLEUKOCYTOSIS

Leukocytosis refers to an increase in the total number of white blood cells in circulation. By definition it is an elevation greater than two standard deviations above the mean circulating white blood cell count based on the age.[57] Hyperleukocytosis is an extreme elevation of the blast count or white blood cell count greater than 100,000/mm^3. It occurs in malignant and nonmalignant disorders, especially acute leukemia.[16] Hyperleukocytosis occurs more frequently in acute leukemia than in chronic leukemia, and its incidence ranges from 5% to 13% in adult acute myeloid leukemia (AML) and from 10% to 30% in adult acute lymphoblastic leukemia (ALL).[58–60] Risk factors for hyperleukocytosis include age <1 year, male gender, certain subtypes of leukemia (French-American-British (FAB) Classification M4, M5), and select cytogenetic abnormalities (11q23 rearrangements and the Philadelphia chromosome).[59,61]

Leukocytosis and leukostasis should be considered a medical emergency as the mortality rate may approach 40%.[59] The management of acute hyperleukocytosis and leukostasis involves supportive measures and reducing the number of circulating leukemic blast cells. Patients may also present with tumor lysis syndrome although this is more often seen after therapy for aggressive hematological disorders such as acute leukemia.[62] Tumor lysis syndrome is discussed in detail in a separate article in this volume.

Pathophysiology

The granulocytic and lymphocytic cell lines are routinely measured in the ED. The granulocytic series is primarily involved in phagocytic activities and is derived from a common progenitor cell located in the bone marrow that also gives rise to erythrocytes, megakaryocytes, eosinophils, basophils, and monocytes. Granulocytes are maintained in a series of developmental and storage pools. The most important is the postmitotic storage pool for neutrophils, which represents 15 to 20 times the circulating population and contains metamyelocytes, band neutrophils, and mature neutrophils. The pool can be drawn on as a ready reserve during rapid consumption of granulocytes. Cytokines and complement components release granulocytes from the marrow storage pool into the circulation, which can result in a two- to threefold increase in the granulocyte count within 4 to 5 hours.[16,57] Circulating neutrophils are subdivided equally into the circulating neutrophil pool and the marginal pool. The marginal pool consists of mature cells adherent to the blood vessel walls, which can rapidly enter the circulating pool and can cause a doubling of the WBC count.[63]

A leukemoid reaction is an excessive leukocytic response in the peripheral blood of the granulocytic cell line. The WBC exceeds 50,000/mm^3 and resembles chronic myeloid leukemia.[64] A leukemoid reaction is characterized by a significant increase in neutrophils in the peripheral blood and a differential demonstrating a left shift.[65] The precursors (myelocytes, metamyelocytes, promyelocytes, and myeloblasts) may occasionally be observed in severe reactions. In contrast to acute leukemia, proliferation and orderly maturation of all normal myeloid elements is observed in the bone marrow and the morphology of the myeloid elements is normal.[57] Diagnosis of a leukemoid reaction should only be made after excluding a hematologic malignancy.[64]

The morbidity of hyperleukocytosis results primarily from the leukostasis syndrome caused by the increased viscosity and sluggish flow of circulating leukemic blasts in tissue microvasculature.[66–68] A postulated mechanism suggests an increase in blood viscosity and blockade of the microcirculation resulting in organ damage.[58] More recent evidence suggests that interactions between leukemic blasts and the surface of endothelial cells might be responsible for the aggregation in the microcirculation.[59,69] Increased production of cytokines and expression of adhesion markers such as ICAM-1, VCAM-1, and selectin by endothelial cells enables myeloblasts to recruit additional myeloblasts.[69,70] This forms a vicious cycle in which increasingly more cells are trapped in the microcirculation.[69]

Diagnosis

A unique problem with white blood cell disorders is the wide variability of normal quantitative values. Total WBC and neutrophil count in neonates younger than 1 week are physiologically higher than those in older children and adults; however, young infants less than 3 months old have smaller storage pools of neutrophils.[71] The proportion of lymphocytes and absolute lymphocyte counts in children are higher than those in adults. Failure to recognize age-specific lymphocytosis may lead to unnecessary investigations.

Clinical Presentation

In general, leukostasis is observed in AML if the WBC is >100 × 10^9/L and in ALL if the WBC is >400 × 10^9/L.[72–74] Leukostasis is usually associated with a high number of circulating blasts but has also been described with blast counts less than 50,000/mm^3.[75] Hyperleukocytosis is seen in up to 13% of patients with AML, is less common in ALL, and even less common in chronic myeloid leukemia (CML) and chronic lymphocytic leukemia (CLL).[58] The frequency of complications is higher in AML than in ALL because the myeloblasts are larger and more adhesive than lymphoblasts. Leukostasis is present in 12% of adult patients with CML and in up to 60% of pediatric cases, but CML represents only 2% to 7% of childhood leukemias.[76]

The manifestations of acute hyperleukocytosis are protean (**Box 2**). Fever is common, but can be traced to definitive infection in only a small number of these patients.[65,77] Blood cultures should still be obtained so that infection can be ruled out, because hyperleukocytosis can mimic several viral, bacterial, and fungal syndromes.[64]

The hallmark complication for the lungs is pulmonary leukostasis. Pulmonary symptoms may range from dyspnea and chest pain to adult respiratory distress syndrome respiratory arrest.[62,77] Chest radiography may be normal or may reveal varying degrees of interstitial or alveolar infiltrates with or without pleural effusions.[78,79] Pulmonary leukostasis may be difficult to distinguish from pneumonia, but bronchoalveolar lavage or perfusion lung scanning may be helpful tests.[80] Definitive diagnosis is most often retrospective after clinical response to chemotherapy.[80] Pulmonary leukostasis is the single worst prognostic factor in patients presenting with hyperleukocytosis of either AML or CML in blast crisis.[62,79]

Neurologic manifestations can range from headaches and altered mental status to focal deficits and intracranial hemorrhage.[81–83] Vascular complications involve small, medium, and occasionally larger vessels presenting with either hemorrhage or thrombosis.[84] Disseminated intravascular coagulation occurs in 30% to 40% of patients with AML and in 15 to 25% of patients with ALL.[58,85]

Box 2
Reported clinical manifestations of hyperleukocytosis

Constitutional

    Fever

    Malaise

Cardiopulmonary

    Dyspnea

    Pleuritic or nonpleuritic chest pain

    Respiratory distress or arrest

    Pulmonary leukostasis

Neurologic

    Headache

    Altered mental status

    Mild confusion

    Stupor and coma

    Focal central nervous system

    Hearing loss

    Cranial nerve deficits

    Intracranial hemorrhage

Vascular

    Retinal hemorrhage or renal vein thrombosis

    Myocardial infarction

    Acute limb ischemia

    Disseminated intravascular coagulation

Laboratory Evaluation

Evaluation of an individual with concerning symptoms or an abnormal complete blood cell count should include a chemistry panel to evaluate for hepatic or renal dysfunction, and uric acid, potassium, and phosphate levels. Determination of prothrombin time, activated partial thromboplastin time, fibrin degradation products, and fibrinogen is necessary to evaluate for coagulopathy or disseminated intravascular coagulopathy (DIC). Platelets may have to be counted manually, because a spurious elevation of the automated platelet count can occur due to the presence of fragments of white and red blood cells.[86] ABG samples should be interpreted cautiously in hyperleukocytosis, as spuriously low arterial oxygen tension can result from rapid consumption of plasma oxygen by the markedly increased number of white blood cells.[87] In the presence of an elevated cell or platelet count, spuriously low levels of PaO_2 are believed to reflect dissolved oxygen consumption from the arterial blood gas specimen; this phenomenon is sometimes referred to as "leukocyte larceny."[87] Pulse oximetry may be more useful to accurately assess oxygenation status in the setting of hyperleukocytosis.[87] Ultimately, diagnosis depends on the results of bone marrow aspirate and biopsy, which typically reveal replacement of normal hematopoietic precursors with >25% leukemic blasts. This bone marrow biopsy is usually not performed in the ED.[88]

Treatment

Rapid reduction in the number of circulating blast cells (leukocytoreduction) is fundamental to managing hyperleukocytosis and leukostasis syndrome.[65,72,89] Prompt introduction of chemotherapy remains the mainstay of treatment of acute hyperleukocytosis and leukostasis with leukapheresis as an important adjunct.[59] Hydroxyurea given at dosages of 50 to 100 mg/kg/d in 3 to 4 divided doses has been shown to reduce the leukocyte count by 50% to 60% within 24 to 48 hours. Hydroxyurea should be started at the time of initial diagnosis and continued until the count has decreased to safer levels.[58,90] Specific chemotherapy modalities should be initiated in emergent consultation with hematologists.[91]

Leukapheresis rapidly yields leukoreduction and is the initial treatment of hyperleukocytosis with symptoms.[59,92,93] Leukapheresis involves the removal of circulating cells with re-infusion of leukocyte-poor plasma. Evidenced-based guidelines are lacking on when to initiate leukapheresis but it is usually initiated in patients with symptoms of leukostasis or in patients with AML if the blast count is more than 100 × 10^9/L.[72,93] Clinical leukostasis occurs in fewer than 10% of patients with ALL with WBC counts less than 400 × 10^9/L and is rarely indicated.[59,74] However, children with ALL who have WBC counts more than 400 × 10^9/L have more than a 50% chance of developing central nervous system (CNS) and pulmonary complications and leukapheresis should be strongly considered.[59,74] The goal with leukoreduction is to reduce the count to 50,000/mm^3 or less.[59] Leukapheresis is associated with an increase in short-term survival.[94,95] Leukapheresis requires the placement and maintenance of a central venous catheter, which may cause complications. In addition, leukapheresis requires trained personnel and specialized equipment not readily available in most EDs. In significant incidents of hyperleukocytosis, intravenous hydration and hydroxyurea administration as well as leukapheresis may be required; however, these treatments should be performed in consultation with a hematologist or an oncologist. Direct treatment of the underlying cause is the ultimate therapy.

THROMBOCYTOSIS

Thrombocytosis by definition occurs with platelet counts above the normal reference range of approximately 150 to 500 K.[96] Thrombocytosis that occurs as part of an exaggerated physiologic response or inflammatory state is termed "reactive thrombocytosis" (**Box 3**).[97] The ED provider should attempt to differentiate between benign reactive thrombocytosis and essential thrombocytosis (ET) from an underlying myeloproliferative disorder (MPD) in conjunction with hematologic consultation (**Box 4**). Reactive thrombocytosis accounts for most cases.[98] Children are more likely to display reactive thrombocytosis and adults more than 60 years old are more likely to have MPDs. Thrombosis occurs more often than bleeding in ET and arterial thrombosis is three times more prevalent than venous thrombosis (**Box 5**). Bleeding is more likely in ET if platelet counts exceed 1.5 million, but bleeding and thrombosis may occur simultaneously.[96] Longstanding ET patients, like all MPDs, are at risk of acute leukemic transformation.[99]

Pathophysiology

Megakaryocytic production increases in response to elevated cytokines, growth factors, thrombopoietin, interleukins, and granulocyte-stimulating factors.[100,101]

Box 3
Causes of reactive thrombocytosis

- Trauma
- Infection
- Paraneoplastic malignancies
- Chronic inflammatory diseases – inflammatory bowel disease, rheumatoid arthritis, and others
- Asplenic states
- Acute or chronic blood loss
- Rebound thrombocytosis after chemotherapy-induced thrombocytopenia

---

Occasionally this normal response is excessive, resulting in reactive thrombocytosis.[102] Major bleeding occurs primarily in the gastrointestinal tract. Hemarthrosis, intraocular, urogenital, posttraumatic, and postsurgical bleeding occur less commonly. Epistaxis, gingival, and other mucosal bleeding are usually minor. As platelet counts increase, normal levels of Von Willebrand's factor (VWF) are unable to maintain normal platelet/VWF ratios. Measured ristocetin VWF activity decreases resulting in spontaneous bleeding.[102] Bleeding complications are rare in reactive thrombocytosis because platelet counts in reactive thrombocytosis infrequently exceed 1.5 million and therefore normal platelet/VWF ratios can be maintained.[96]

Diagnosis

In assessing thrombocytosis, it is important that the ED provider recognizes the possible presence of an MPD but it is not critical that the specific MPD is identified. Because all MPDs arise from overlapping genetic and clonal abnormalities, disease manifestations often overlap.[102] Splenomegaly and hepatomegaly may occur in any of the MPDs.[96] Bone marrow and cytogenetic results that indicate underlying clonal abnormalities are supportive of an MPD.[103] JAK2 mutation is also present in ET and it carries a higher risk of thromboembolic events than in patients without the mutation.[104] These patients also exhibit higher red and white cell counts. Acute phase reactants including elevated C-reactive protein (CRP) levels or increased sedimentation rate suggests reactive thrombocytosis.[105] Numerous megakaryocytes, megakaryocytic fragments, or other myeloid precursor cells seen on peripheral blood smear are more consistent with an MPD.[27]

Pseudothrombocytosis occurs if automated blood analyzers cannot distinguish true platelets from amorphous cellular fragments.[106] Pseudothrombocytosis is most commonly seen with extreme leukocytosis (CLL), rapid intravascular hemolysis,

---

Box 4
Causes of thrombocytosis in chronic myeloproliferative disorders

- Essential thrombocytosis (5.5%), ET
- Chronic myeloid leukemia (3.3%), CML
- Polycythemia vera (2.5%), PCV
- Other (1%)

Box 5
Thromboembolic complications of essential thrombosis

- Arterial

   Cerebral

   Upper and lower extremities

   Microcirculatory

- Deep venous thrombosis

   Pelvic mesenteric

   Hepatic portal

   Spleen

   Cerebral sinuses

---

burns, postsplenectomy states (Howell Jolly bodies are also seen) and in the "sticky platelet syndrome."[107] If thrombocytosis is present, serum potassium levels will be elevated (pseudohyperkalemia) due to the degranulation of platelets in vitro; however, the more accurate plasma potassium levels will be normal.[108]

Prognosis

Platelet counts are not a reliable predictor of thrombosis in any individual patient with essential thrombocytosis, although platelet counts higher than 600 K are generally associated with an increased risk of thrombosis.[98] Thrombohemorragic risk is negligible in cases of clear reactive thrombocytosis without underlying MPD.[98] Patients with a possible underlying MPD are considered low risk if they are <60 years old, have no symptoms or history of a thromboembolic or hemorrhagic event, and platelet counts are less than 1.5 million.[109,110] Reactive thrombocytosis and select low-risk MPD patients can be safely managed as outpatients.[98]

Treatment

Treatment of ET in intermediate- and high-risk groups includes aspirin and hydroxyurea.[96,102,109,111] Hydroxyurea reduces massive splenomegaly, and can be added to aspirin therapy to decrease microvascular symptoms in resistant cases.[102] Short-term side effects include neutropenia, macrocytic anemia, nausea, vomiting, diarrhea, skin ulcerations, and teratogenicity.[96,109] The greatest concern with hydroxyurea is the risk of leukemic transformation, so long-term therapy decisions should be referred to specialists.[109] Sudden withdrawal of hydoxyurea can result in a rebound thrombocytosis and doses must be reduced in the presence of renal insufficiency. Interferon alpha is best reserved for pregnant patients with thrombocytosis and a known MPD.[96] Since 2005, anagrelide, a platelet-reducing drug that decreases megakaryocyte maturation has fallen out of favor due to evidence of unacceptable risks and superiority of hydroxyurea.[111,112] Treatment of acute major thrombotic or bleeding events also includes hydroxyurea, interferon alpha in pregnant patients, and emergent platelet pheresis.

SUMMARY

The myeloproliferative disorders and the hyperviscosity syndrome can rapidly manifest with emergent presentations. Emergency medicine providers should be aware of these conditions and be prepared to rapidly initiate supportive and early definitive management including plasma exchange and apharesis. Early consultation with a hematologist is essential for management of this complex patient population.

REFERENCES

1. Bekelman J, Jackson N, Donehower RC. Oncologic emergencies. In: Nilsson KR, Piccini JP, editors. The Osler medical handbook. 2nd edition. Philadelphia: Saunders Elsevier; 2006.
2. Zojer N, Ludwig H. Hematological emergencies. Ann Oncol 2007;1(Suppl 18): i45–8.
3. Frewin R, Henson A, Provan D. ABC of clinical haematology. Haematological emergencies. BMJ 1997;314(7090):1333–6.
4. Mehta J, Singhal S. Hyperviscosity syndrome in plasma cell dyscrasias. Semin Thromb Hemost 2003;29(5):467–71.
5. Nkwuo N, Schamban N, Borenstein M. Selected oncologic emergencies. In: Marx JA, editor. Rosen's emergency medicine: concepts and clinical practice. Philadelphia: Mosby; 2006.
6. Vijay A, Gertz MA. Waldenstrom macroglobulinemia. Blood 2007;109(12): 5096–103.
7. Rajkumar VS, Dispenzieri AS, Kyle RA. Monoclonal gammopathy of undetermined significance, Waldenstrom macroglobulinemia, AL amyloidosis, and related plasma cell disorders: diagnosis and treatment. Mayo Clin Proc 2006; 81(5):693–703.
8. McPherson RA, Pincus MR. Henry's clinical diagnosis and management by laboratory methods. 21st edition. Philadelphia: W.B. Saunders; 2006.
9. Mullen EC, Wang M. Recognizing hyperviscosity syndrome in patients with Waldenstrom macroglobulinemia. Clin J Oncol Nurs 2007;11(1):87–95.
10. Shaheen SP, Talwalkar SS, Medeiros LJ, et al. Multiple myeloma and immunosecretory disorders: an update. Adv Anat Pathol 2008;15(4):196–210.
11. Garderet L, Fabiani B, Lacombe K, et al. Hyperviscosity syndrome in an HIV-1-positive patient. Am J Med 2004;117(11):891–3.
12. Chu K, Kang DW, Kim DE, et al. Magnetic resonance findings of hemichorea-hemiballismus associated with diabetic hyperglycemia: a hyperviscosity syndrome? [miscellaneous article]. Arch Neurol 2002;59(3):448–52.
13. Paul B. Polyclonal hypergammaglobulinaemia with hyperviscosity syndrome. Br J Haematol 2002;118(3):922–3.
14. Kesmarky G, Kenyeres P, Rabai M, et al. Plasma viscosity: a forgotten variable. Clin Hemorheol Microcirc 2008;39(1–4):243–6.
15. Rosencranz R, Bogen SA. Clinical laboratory measurement of serum, plasma, and blood viscosity. Am J Clin Pathol 2006;125(Suppl):S78–86.
16. Winters JL, Pineda AA. Hemapheresis. In: McPherson RA, Pincus MR, editors. Henry's clinical diagnosis and management by laboratory methods. 21st editon. Philadelphia: W.B. Saunders Company; 2006.
17. Ramsakal A, Beaupre D. Cancer emergencies: hyperviscosity syndromes. In: Williams MV, editor. Comprehensive hospital medicine. Philadelphia: Saunders; 2007.
18. Eby C, Blinder M. Hemostatic complications associated with paraproteinemias. Curr Hematol Rep 2003;2(5):388–94.
19. Menke MN, Feke GT, McMeel JW, et al. Hyperviscosity-related retinopathy in Waldenstrom macroglobulinemia. Arch Ophthalmol 2006;124(11):1601–6.

20. Syms MJ, Arcila ME, Holtel MR. Waldenstrom's macroglobulinemia and sensorineural hearing loss. Am J Otol 2001;22(5):349–53.

21. Vitolo U, Ferreri AJ, Montoto S, et al. Lymphoplasmacytic lymphoma – Waldenstrom's macroglobulinemia. Crit Rev Oncol Hematol 2008;67(2):172–85.

22. Higdon ML, Higdon JA. Treatment of oncologic emergencies. Am Fam Physician 2006;74(11):1873–80.

23. Burwick N, Roccaro AM, Leleu X, et al. Targeted therapies in Waldenstrom macroglobulinemia. Curr Opin Investig Drugs 2008;9(6):631–7.

24. Goldschmidt H, Lannert H, Bommer J, et al. Multiple myeloma and renal failure. Nephrol Dial Transplant 2000;15(3):301–4.

25. Dimopoulos MA, Kastritis E, Rosinol L, et al. Pathogenesis and treatment of renal failure in multiple myeloma. Leukemia 2008;22(8):1485–93.

26. Sharma BD, Kabra SR, Gupta B. Symmetrical peripheral gangrene. Trop Doct 2004;34(1):2–4.

27. Bain BJ. Diagnosis from the blood smear. N Engl J Med 2005;353(5):498–507.

28. Weinstein R, Mahmood M. Case 6-2002– a 54-year-old woman with left, then right, central-retinal-vein occlusion. N Engl J Med 2002;346(8):603–10.

29. McKenna JA. Waldenstrom's macroglobulinemia. Clin J Oncol Nurs 2002;6(5): 283–6.

30. Teruya J. Practical issues in therapeutic apheresis. Ther Apher 2002;6(4):288–9.

31. Johnson SA. Advances in the treatment of Waldenstrom's macroglobulinemia. Expert Rev Anticancer Ther 2006;6(3):329–34.

32. Tefferi A. Essential thrombocythemia, polycythemia vera, and myelofibrosis: current management and the prospect of targeted therapy. Am J Hematol 2008;83(6):491–7.

33. Prchal JT. Polycythemia vera and other primary polycythemias. Curr Opin Hematol 2005;12(2):112–6.

34. Lorberboym M, Rahimi-Levene N, Lipszyc H, et al. Analysis of red cell mass and plasma volume in patients with polycythemia. Arch Pathol Lab Med 2005;129(1): 89–91.

35. Dams K, Meersseman W, Verbeken E, et al. A 59-year-old man with shock, polycythemia, and an underlying paraproteinemia. Chest 2007;132(4):1393–6.

36. Tefferi A, Spivak JL. Polycythemia vera: scientific advances and current practice. Semin Hematol 2005;42(4):206–20.

37. Lippert E, Boissinot M, Kralovics R, et al. The JAK2-V617F mutation is frequently present at diagnosis in patients with essential thrombocythemia and polycythemia vera. Blood 2006;108(6):1865–7.

38. Scott LM, Tong W, Levine RL, et al. JAK2 exon 12 mutations in polycythemia vera and idiopathic erythrocytosis. N Engl J Med 2007;356(5): 459–68.

39. Schafer AI. Molecular basis of the diagnosis and treatment of polycythemia vera and essential thrombocythemia. Blood 2006;107(11):4214–22.

40. Halperin ML, Cheema-Dhadli S, Lin SH, et al. Properties permitting the renal cortex to be the oxygen sensor for the release of erythropoietin: clinical implications. Clin J Am Soc Nephrol 2006;1(5):1049–53.

41. Hodges VM, Rainey S, Lappin TR, et al. Pathophysiology of anemia and erythrocytosis. Crit Rev Oncol Hematol 2007;64(2):139–58.

42. Takeda K, Aguila HL, Parikh NS, et al. Regulation of adult erythropoiesis by prolyl hydroxylase domain proteins. Blood 2008;111(6):3229–35.

43. Finazzi G, Gregg XT, Barbui T, et al. Idiopathic erythrocytosis and other nonclonal polycythemias. Best Pract Res Clin Haematol 2006;19(3):471–82.

44. Mossuz P, Girodon F, Donnard M, et al. Diagnostic value of serum erythropoietin level in patients with absolute erythrocytosis. Haematologica 2004;89(10):1194–8.
45. Spivak JL, Silver RT. The revised World Health Organization diagnostic criteria for polycythemia vera, essential thrombocytosis, and primary myelofibrosis: an alternative proposal. Blood 2008;112(2):231–9.
46. Prchal JT, Pastore YD. Erythropoietin and erythropoiesis: polycythemias due to disruption of oxygen homeostasis. Hematol J 2004;5(Suppl 3):S110–3.
47. Gordeuk VR, Prchal JT. Vascular complications in Chuvash polycythemia. Semin Thromb Hemost 2006;32(3):289–94.
48. Gordeuk VR, Stockton DW, Prchal JT. Congenital polycythemias/erythrocytoses. Haematologica 2005;90(1):109–16.
49. Lee Y-S, Vortmeyer AO, Lubensky IA, et al. Coexpression of erythropoietin and erythropoietin receptor in von Hippel-Lindau disease-associated renal cysts and renal cell carcinoma. Clin Cancer Res 2005;11(3):1059–64.
50. Windsor JS, Rodway GW. Heights and haematology: the story of haemoglobin at altitude. Postgrad Med J 2007;83(977):148–51.
51. Tefferi A, Thiele J, Orazi A, et al. Proposals and rationale for revision of the World Health Organization diagnostic criteria for polycythemia vera, essential thrombocythemia, and primary myelofibrosis: recommendations from an ad hoc international expert panel. Blood 2007;110(4):1092–7.
52. Tefferi A, Vardiman JW. Classification and diagnosis of myeloproliferative neoplasms: the 2008 World Health Organization criteria and point-of-care diagnostic algorithms. Leukemia 2007;22(1):14–22.
53. Landolfi R, Marchioli R, Kutti J, et al. Efficacy and safety of low-dose aspirin in polycythemia vera. N Engl J Med 2004;350(2):114–24.
54. Finazzi G, Barbui T. How I treat patients with polycythemia vera. Blood 2007; 109(12):5104–11.
55. Tefferi A. Polycythemias. In: Goldman L, Ausiello D, editors. Cecil's medicine. 23rd edition. Philadelphia: Saunders; 2007.
56. Hamilton GC, Janz TJ. Anemia, polycythemia, and white blood cell disorders. In: Marx JA, editor. Rosen's emergency medicine: concepts and clinical practice. Philadelphia: Mosby; 2006.
57. Hoffman R, Benz EJ, Shattil SJ, et al. Hematology: basic principles and practice. Philadelphia: Elsevier; 2005.
58. Porcu P, Cripe LD, Ng EW, et al. Hyperleukocytic leukemias and leukostasis: a review of pathophysiology, clinical presentation and management. Leuk Lymphoma 2000;39(1–2):1–18.
59. Porcu P, Farag S, Marcucci G, et al. Leukocytoreduction for acute leukemia. Ther Apher 2002;6(1):15–23.
60. Nowacki P, Zdziarska B, Fryze C, et al. Co-existence of thrombocytopenia and hyperleukocytosis ('critical period') as a risk factor of haemorrhage into the central nervous system in patients with acute leukaemias. Haematologia 2002; 31(4):347–55.
61. Pui CH, Robison LL, Look AT, et al. Acute lymphoblastic leukaemia. Lancet 2008;371(9617):1030–43.
62. Leis JF, Primack SL, Schubach SE, et al. Management of life-threatening pulmonary leukostasis with single agent imatinib mesylate during CML myeloid blast crisis. Haematologica 2004;89(9):102–3.
63. Hamilton G, Janz T. Anemia, polycythemia, and white blood cell disorders. In: Rosen P, editor. Emergency medicine concepts and clinical practice. Philadelphia: Mosby; 2006. p. 1867–91.

64. Sakka V, Tsiodras S, Giamarellos-Bourboulis EJ, et al. An update on the etiology and diagnostic evaluation of a leukemoid reaction. Eur J Intern Med 2006;17(6): 394–8.
65. Halfdanarson TR, Hogan WJ, Moynihan TJ, et al. Oncologic emergencies: diagnosis and treatment. Mayo Clin Proc 2006;81(6):835–48.
66. Kwaan H, Vicuna B. Thrombosis and bleeding in cancer patients. Oncology Review 2007;1(1):14–27.
67. Lawrence YR, Raveh D, Rudensky B, et al. Extreme leukocytosis in the emergency department. QJM 2007;100(4):217–23.
68. Sadeghi-Nejad H, Dogra V, Seftel AD, et al. Priapism. Radiol Clin North Am 2004;42(2):427–43.
69. Stucki A, Rivier AS, Gikic M, et al. Endothelial cell activation by myeloblasts: molecular mechanisms of leukostasis and leukemic cell dissemination. Blood 2001;97(7):2121–9.
70. Zhang W, Zhang X, Fan X, et al. Effect of ICAM-1 and LFA-1 in hyperleukocytic acute myeloid leukaemia. Clin Lab Haematol 2006;28(3):177–82.
71. Athale UH, Chan AK. Hemorrhagic complications in pediatric hematologic malignancies. Semin Thromb Hemost 2007;33(4):408–15.
72. Majhail NS, Lichtin AE. Acute leukemia with a very high leukocyte count: confronting a medical emergency. Cleve Clin J Med 2004;71(8):633–7.
73. Marbello L, Ricci F, Nosari AM, et al. Outcome of hyperleukocytic adult acute myeloid leukaemia: a single-center retrospective study and review of literature. Leuk Res 2008;32(8):1221–7.
74. Szczepiorkowski ZM, Bandarenko N, Kim HC, et al. Guidelines on the use of therapeutic apheresis in clinical practice: evidence-based approach from the Apheresis Applications Committee of the American Society for Apheresis. J Clin Apheresis 2007;22(3):106–75.
75. Buchem MA, Velde J, Willemze R, et al. Leucostasis, an underestimated cause of death in leukaemia. Ann Hematol 1988;56(1):39–44.
76. Rowe JM, Lichtman MA. Hyperleukocytosis and leukostasis: common features of childhood chronic myelogenous leukemia. Blood 1984;63(5):1230–4.
77. Wu YK, Huang YC, Huang SF, et al. Acute respiratory distress syndrome caused by leukemic infiltration of the lung. J Formos Med Assoc 2008;107(5):419–23.
78. Azoulay E, Fieux F, Moreau D, et al. Acute monocytic leukemia presenting as acute respiratory failure. Am J Respir Crit Care Med 2003;167(10):1329–33.
79. Szyper-Kravitz M, Strahilevitz J, Oren V, et al. Pulmonary leukostasis: role of perfusion lung scan in diagnosis and follow up. Am J Hematol 2001;67(2):136–8.
80. Ezzie ME, Mastronarde J. Refractory hypoxia secondary to pulmonary leukostasis treated successfully with irradiation. Chest 2006;130(4):332S–3S.
81. Kim H, Lee JH, Choi SJ, et al. Analysis of fatal intracranial hemorrhage in 792 acute leukemia patients. Haematologica 2004;89(5):622–4.
82. Tsai CC, Huang CB, Sheen JM, et al. Sudden hearing loss as the initial manifestation of chronic myeloid leukemia in a child. Chang Gung Med J 2004;27(8): 629–33.
83. Hsu WH, Chu SJ, Tsai WC, et al. Acute myeloid leukemia presenting as one-and-a-half syndrome. Am J Emerg Med 2008;26(4):513, e511–2.
84. Cukierman T, Gatt ME, Libster D, et al. Chronic lymphocytic leukemia presenting with extreme hyperleukocytosis and thrombosis of the common femoral vein. Leuk Lymphoma 2002;43(9):1865–8.
85. Tallman MS, Kwaan HC. Intravascular clotting activation and bleeding in patients with hematologic malignancies. Rev Clin Exp Hematol 2004;8(1):E1.

86. Li S, Salhany KE. Spurious elevation of automated platelet counts in secondary acute monocytic leukemia associated with tumor lysis syndrome. Arch Pathol Lab Med 1999;123(11):1111–4.
87. Lele AV, Mirski MA, Stevens RD, et al. Spurious hypoxemia. Crit Care Med 2005; 33(8):1854–6.
88. Kolitz JE. Acute leukemia in children. In: Rakel R, Bope E, editors. Conn's current therapy. Philadelphia: Elsevier; 2008. p. 446–53.
89. Dutcher JP, Schiffer CA, Wiernik PH. Hyperleukocytosis in adult acute nonlymphocytic leukemia: impact on remission rate and duration, and survival. J Clin Oncol 1987;5(9):1364–72.
90. Kasner MT, Laury A, Kasner SE, et al. Increased cerebral blood flow after leukapheresis for acute myelogenous leukemia. Am J Hematol 2007;82(12): 1110–2.
91. Lo-Coco F, Ammatuna E. Front line clinical trials and minimal residual disease monitoring in acute promyelocytic leukemia. Curr Top Microbiol Immunol 2007;313:145–56.
92. Blum W, Porcu P. Therapeutic apheresis in hyperleukocytosis and hyperviscosity syndrome. Semin Thromb Hemost 2007;33(4):350–4.
93. Zarkovic M, Kwaan HC. Correction of hyperviscosity by apheresis. Semin Thromb Hemost 2003;29(5):535–42.
94. Thiebaut A, Thomas X, Belhabri A, et al. Impact of pre-induction therapy leukapheresis on treatment outcome in adult acute myelogenous leukemia presenting with hyperleukocytosis. Ann Hematol 2000;79(9):501–6.
95. Bug G, Anargyrou K, Tonn T, et al. Impact of leukapheresis on early death rate in adult acute myeloid leukemia presenting with hyperleukocytosis. Transfusion 2007;47(10):1843–50.
96. Schafer AI. Thrombocytosis. N Engl J Med 2004;350(12):1211–9.
97. Keung YK, Owen J. Iron deficiency and thrombosis: literature review. Clin Appl Thromb Hemost 2004;10(4):387–91.
98. Vannucchi AM, Barbui T. Thrombocytosis and thrombosis. Hematology 2007; 2007(1):363–70.
99. Chomienne C, Rain JD, Briere J, et al. Risk of leukemic transformation in PV and ET patients. Pathol Biol 2004;52(5):289–93.
100. Spivak JL. The chronic myeloproliferative disorders: clonality and clinical heterogeneity. Semin Hematol 2004;41(2 Suppl 3):1–5.
101. Sierko E, Wojtukiewicz MZ. Platelets and angiogenesis in malignancy. Semin Thromb Hemost 2004;30(1):95–108.
102. Tefferi A. Essential thrombocythemia: scientific advances and current practice. Curr Opin Hematol 2006;13(2):93–8.
103. Thiele J, Kvasnicka HM, Diehl V. Standardization of bone marrow features – does it work in hematopathology for histological discrimination of different disease patterns? Histol Histopathol 2005;20(2):633–44.
104. Levine RL, Gilliland DG. JAK-2 mutations and their relevance to myeloproliferative disease. Curr Opin Hematol 2007;14(1):43–7.
105. Powner DJ, Hoots WK. Thrombocytosis in the NICU. Neurocrit Care 2008;8(3): 471–5.
106. van der Meer W, MacKenzie MA, Dinnissen JWB, et al. Pseudoplatelets: a retrospective study of their incidence and interference with platelet counting. J Clin Pathol 2003;56(10):772–4.
107. Frenkel EP, Mammen EF. Sticky platelet syndrome and thrombocythemia. Hematol Oncol Clin North Am 2003;17(1):63–83.

108. Sevastos N, Theodossiades G, Efstathiou S, et al. Pseudohyperkalemia in serum: the phenomenon and its clinical magnitude. J Lab Clin Med 2006; 147(3):139–44.
109. Briere JB. Essential thrombocythemia. Orphanet J Rare Dis 2007;2:3.
110. Kessler CM. Propensity for hemorrhage and thrombosis in chronic myeloproliferative disorders. Semin Hematol 2004;41(2 Suppl 3):10–4.
111. Harrison CN, Campbell PJ, Buck G, et al. Hydroxyurea compared with anagrelide in high-risk essential thrombocythemia. N Engl J Med 2005;353(1):33–45.
112. Dingli D, Tefferi A. A critical review of anagrelide therapy in essential thrombocythemia and related disorders. Leuk Lymphoma 2005;46(5):641–50.
113. Barosi G, Mesa RA, Thiele J, et al. Proposed criteria for the diagnosis of post-polycythemia vera and post-essential thrombocythemia myelofibrosis: a consensus statement from the International Working Group for Myelofibrosis Research and Treatment. Leukemia 2008;22(2):437–8.

Management of Acquired Bleeding Problems in Cancer Patients

Thomas G. DeLoughery, MD[a,b,c],*

KEYWORDS
- Bleeding • Cancer • Leukemia • Myeloma • Amyloid
- Disseminated intravascular coagulation

APPROACH TO THE BLEEDING CANCER PATIENT

Patient Review

Patients with underlying cancer can present to the Emergency Department (ED) with bleeding related to the underlying malignancy, antineoplastic treatment, or nonmalignancy-related factors. No matter how extreme the situation, the ED physician should try to obtain a complete history about the patient including therapies that they have recently received. In additional, the physical examination can provide valuable clues. For example, the presence of multiple sites of diffuse bleeding signals the presence of coagulopathy such as disseminated intravascular coagulation (DIC). The appearance of multiple ecchymotic lesions should alert the clinician to consider purpura fulminans.

Laboratories

The first step in evaluation of any bleeding patient is to obtain a basic set of coagulation tests. The international normalized ratio (INR) activated partial thromboplastin time (aPTT), platelet count, and fibrinogen level can be obtained rapidly. Three patterns of defects can be seen in the INR and aPTT (**Box 1**). Isolated elevations of the INR indicate a factor VII deficiency. In sick patients, low factor VII levels are also

A version of this article was previously published in the *Emergency Medicine Clinics of North America*, 27:3.

[a] Divisions of Hematology and Medical Oncology, Department of Medicine, L586, Oregon Health & Science University, 3181 SW Sam Jackson Park Road, Portland, OR 97201-3098, USA

[b] Division of Laboratory Medicine, Department of Pathology, Oregon Health & Science University, 3181 SW Sam Jackson Park Road, Portland, OR 97201-3098, USA

[c] Divisions of Hematology and Medical Oncology, Department of Pediatrics, Oregon Health & Science University, 3181 SW Sam Jackson Park Road, Portland, OR 97201-3098, USA

* Divisions of Hematology and Medical Oncology, Department of Medicine, L586, Oregon Health & Science University, 3181 SW Sam Jackson Park Road, Portland, OR 97201-3098.

E-mail address: delought@ohsu.edu

Box 1
Interpretation of coagulation tests

Elevated prothrombin time, normal aPTT

Factor VII deficiency

    Vitamin K deficiency

    Warfarin

    Sepsis

Normal prothrombin time, elevated aPTT

Isolated factor deficiency (VIII, IX, XI, XII, contact pathway proteins)

Specific factor inhibitor

Heparin

Lupus inhibitor

Elevated prothrombin time, elevated aPTT

Multiple coagulation factor deficiencies

    Liver disease

    Disseminated intravascular coagulation (DIC)

Isolated factor X, V or II deficiency

Factor V inhibitors

High hematocrits (>60% spurious)

High heparin levels

Severe vitamin K deficiency

Low fibrinogen (<50 mg/dL)

Dysfibrinogemia

Dilutional

---

common due to third spacing and increased consumption leading to an elevated INR.[1] A marked elevation of the INR out of proportion to the aPTT suggests vitamin K deficiency. Isolated elevation of the aPTT has many causes. Prolongation of the INR and aPTT suggests multiple defects or deficiency of factors II, V, or X, and marked prolongation of the INR and aPTT can also be seen with low levels of fibrinogen. Further coagulation tests should be ordered based on the INR and aPTT to better define the defect if the reason for the coagulation deficiency is not apparent from the history. Ideally, these tests should be done in conjunction with a hematology consultant.

If the platelet count is low, examination of the blood smear by the laboratory technician is essential to make sure that the artifact of platelet clumping (pseudothrombocytopenia) is not present. Although many processes can cause a moderately low platelet count, the differential diagnosis for isolated profound thrombocytopenia (<10,000/μL) is generally limited to immune thrombocytopenia, drug-induced thrombocytopenia, or post–transfusion purpura.

Excessive bleeding has been reported with plasma fibrinogen levels less than 50 mg/dL. The end points of the INR and aPTT are timed to the formation of the fibrin clot. If plasma levels of fibrinogen decrease to less than 80 mg/dL, the clot may be small and not detected by the machine, resulting in a prolonged INR and aPTT. Low fibrinogen levels reflect severe liver disease, consumptive coagulopathy, or dilution by infusion of massive amounts of resuscitative fluids.

Some bleeding disorders, such as platelet function defects or increases in fibrinolysis, cannot be detected by routine laboratory tests. Performing rapid tests to assess platelet function remains controversial. Bleeding times are difficult to perform in the ED and are not predictive of bleeding risk.[2] The PFA–100 is a rapid automatic test for platelet function that is likely to replace the bleeding time, but there are no data on the use of this rapid test to guide therapy for acute bleeding in the ED.[3] It is also difficult to assess for excessive fibrinolysis. The euglobulin clot lysis time is a screen for fibrinolysis but it is not standardized and can be difficult to obtain. Thromboelastography is a unique point-of-care laboratory test that examines whole blood thrombus formation and lysis, but it is not widely available and requires experience in interpretation.[4]

MASSIVE TRANSFUSION THERAPY

Acute bleeding in cancer patients can require large amounts of transfusion products. Early data showed high mortality rates with transfusion of more than 20 units of blood.[5] With modern blood bank techniques and improved laboratory testing, survival rates of 43% to 70% are achieved in patients transfused with more than 50 units of blood.

The approach to massive transfusions is to measure the five basic laboratory tests outlined in **Box 2** These tests reflect the fundamental parameters essential for blood volume and hemostasis. Current recommended replacement therapy is based on the results of these tests and the clinical situation of the patient. With rapid transfusion devices, a unit of product can be given in minutes. After infusing the initial blood products, the basic laboratories test should be repeated to guide additional therapy. The transfusion threshold for a low hematocrit depends on the stability of the patient. If the hematocrit is less than 30% and the patient is bleeding or hemodynamically unstable, packed red cells should be transfused. Stable patients can tolerate a lower hematocrit; an aggressive transfusion policy may even be detrimental.[6]

If the patient is actively bleeding, has florid DIC, or has received platelet aggregation inhibitors, then keeping the platelet count above 50,000/μL is reasonable because this

---

Box 2
Massive transfusions

The five basic tests of hemostasis

Hematocrit

Platelet count

Prothrombin time (PT-INR)

Activated partial thromboplastin time (aPTT)

Fibrinogen level

Management guidelines

1. Platelets <50 to 75,000/μL: give 1 plateletpheresis concentrate or 6 to 8 packs of single donor platelets

2. Fibrinogen <125 mg/dL: give 10 units of cryoprecipitate

3. Hematocrit less than 30%: give red cells

4. Prothrombin time INR >2.0 and aPTT abnormal: give 2 to 4 units of fresh frozen plasma (FFP).

results in less microvascular bleeding.[7] The conventional dose of platelets is six to eight platelet concentrates or one plateletpheresis unit.

For a fibrinogen level of less than 100 mg/dL, transfusion of 10 units of cryoprecipitate will increase the plasma fibrinogen level by approximately 100 mg/dL. In certain clinical situations, such as acute promyelocytic leukemia, severe fibrinolysis can occur, and the need for large amounts of cryoprecipitate should be anticipated.

In patients with an INR greater than two and an abnormal aPTT, two to four units of fresh frozen plasma (FFP) can be given. For an aPTT greater than 1.5 times normal, two to four units of plasma should be given. Patients with marked abnormalities such as an aPTT twice normal may require aggressive therapy with at least 15 to 30 mL/kg (4–8 units for an average adult) of plasma.[8]

Occasionally, empirical transfusion therapy for the severely bleeding patient is required. Platelet products should be given first because they will also provide plasma replacement. In patients also likely to have DIC (eg, leukemia), administration of 10 units of cryoprecipitate is indicated. For patients who are likely to receive 10 or more units of blood, early use of FFP may help preserve coagulation.[9] One approach is to thaw the plasma and give four units whenever six or more units of uncrossmatched blood are given to a patient with massive bleeding. Recent studies suggest that matching 1:1 units of RBC and FFP may improve outcomes.[10]

Complications of Transfusions

Hypothermia commonly complicates the care of massively transfused patients and can worsen bleeding.[11] Hypothermia impairs platelet function, decreases the efficiency of coagulation reactions, and enhances fibrinolysis. Unwarmed packed red cells can lower the body temperature by 0.25°C.[12] Hypothermia can be prevented by transfusion of blood through blood warmers. Electrolyte abnormalities are unusual even after massive transfusion. Platelet concentrates and plasma contains citrate, which can chelate calcium. However, the citrate is rapidly metabolized and clinically significant hypocalcemia is rare. Although empirical calcium replacement is often recommended, one study suggests that its use is associated with a worse outcome.[13] If hypocalcemia is a clinical concern, then ionized calcium levels should be monitored to guide therapy.

Although potassium leaks out of stored red cells, even older units of blood only contain a total of 8 mEq/L of potassium, so hyperkalemia is not usually a concern. Stored blood is acidic with a pH of 6.5 to 6.9, but acidosis attributed solely to transfused blood is rare. Empirical bicarbonate replacement has been associated with severe alkalosis and is not recommended.[14]

Recombinant Factor VIIa

Recombinant factor VIIa (rVIIa) was originally developed as a bypass agent to support hemostasis in hemophiliacs with inhibitors.[15] Recently, there has been an explosion of information concerning rVIIa use for a wide array of bleeding disorders.[16] Increasingly, rVIIa is being used as a universal hemostatic agent for patients with uncontrolled bleeding from any mechanism. Multiple case reports have demonstrated successful use of rVIIa for bleeding in cardiac surgery patients, obstetric bleeding, reversal of anticoagulation, and trauma. Unfortunately, a paucity of prospective data exists to put these anecdotes into recommended clinical practice.[17]

A general approach for use of rVIIa for acute bleeding would be to first ensure that a reasonable attempt has been made to correct coagulation status, and that there is a defined, survivable condition.[16] Although dosing recommendations vary, a reasonable dose of rVIIa for most situations is 90 μg/kg. If hemostasis is not obtained within 30 minutes, there is little use in giving a second dose. If the patient improves and then rebleeds after 2 to 3 hours, another dose can be given.

Although hypothermia has a detrimental effect on blood coagulation, this does not seem to affect the function of rVIIa. In vitro studies show no decrease in the effect of rVIIa on thrombin generation at 33°C and this finding is supported by clinical data.[18] In contrast, low pH does seem to have a negative effect. In vitro, the effect of rVIIa was reduced by 90% when the pH was lowered from 7.4 to 7.0, which is also supported by clinical data showing that trauma patients who did not respond to rVIIa were more likely to have pH less than 7.2 compared with responders.[19] This finding supports the idea of aggressive resuscitation before resorting to rVIIa.

In theory, rVIIa-induced coagulation activation would be expected to result in DIC or overwhelming thrombosis, but thrombotic complications are rare. In 700,000 doses given to hemophiliacs, only 16 thrombotic complications were seen.[20] However, if used in older patients, especially those with vascular risk factors, the risk of arterial thrombosis seems to increase.[21] In the trials for intracranial hemorrhage, the thrombosis rate after use of rVIIa was 5% to 9%.[22] This risk may be augmented by the known prothrombotic state of cancer. Until more safety data are available, the risk/benefit ratio should be considered before using rVIIa in cancer patients, especially in those with a history of vascular disease such as strokes or myocardial infarction.

COAGULATION FACTOR-RELATED BLEEDING
Acquired Von Willebrand Disease

Acquired von Willebrand disease (VWD) occurs in lymphomas, myeloproliferative syndromes, myeloma, and monoclonal gammopathies.[23,24] The most common presentations are diffuse oozing from surgical sites, the nose, or gastrointestinal bleeding.[25] Patients with acquired VWD can present as type 1 (decreased protein) or type 2 (abnormal protein) disease.[26]

Patients with acquired VWD have variable responses to therapy.[23,27] Desmopressin is effective in many patients with acquired VWD types 1 and 2 but, consistent with the antibody-mediated destruction, the magnitude and duration of the effect is often reduced.[28] For bleeding patients, high doses of the von Willebrand concentrate Humate−P are indicated.[29] For patients with strong inhibitors that factor concentrates cannot overcome or with life-threatening bleeding, rVIIa may prove useful.[30]

Acquired Factor VIII Inhibitors

Factor VIII deficiency due to autoantibodies is the most frequent acquired coagulation factor deficiency complication in older cancer patients.[31] Unlike classic hemophiliacs, these patients often have ecchymoses covering large areas of their body, and can have massive muscle and soft tissue bleeding. Patients will have prolonged aPTTs, a positive test for an inhibitor, and a low factor VIII level. For severe or life-threatening bleeding, recombinant VIIa is the treatment of choice.[32] The dose is 90 μg/kg repeated every 2 to 3 hours until bleeding has stopped.

Disseminated Intravascular Coagulation

DIC is the clinical manifestation of inappropriate thrombin activation.[33] The activation of thrombin leads to (1) fibrinogen conversion to fibrin, (2) platelet activation and consumption, (3) factors V and VIII activation, (4) protein C activation (and degradation of factors Va and VIIIa), (5) endothelial cell activation, and (6) fibrinolysis.

Patients with DIC can present in 1 of 4 patterns:

1) Asymptomatic: patients can present with laboratory evidence of DIC but no bleeding or thrombosis (often seen in patients with sepsis or cancer). However, with further progression of the underlying disease, these patients can rapidly become symptomatic.
2) Bleeding: bleeding is due to a combination of factor depletion, platelet dysfunction, thrombocytopenia, and excessive fibrinolysis. These patients may present with diffuse bleeding from multiple sites.
3) Thrombosis: despite the general activation of the coagulation process, thrombosis is unusual in most patients with acute DIC. An exception to this is cancer patients in whom thrombosis can be the major complicating factor. Most often the thrombosis is venous, but arterial thrombosis and nonbacterial thrombotic endocarditis have been reported.
4) Purpura fulminans, which is DIC in association with symmetric limb ecchymosis and necrosis of the skin, is seen in two situations.[34] Primary purpura fulminans is most often seen after a viral infection such as varicella in an immunocompromised child. In these patients the purpura fulminans starts with a painful red area on an extremity that rapidly progresses to a black ischemic area. Secondary purpura fulminans is most often associated with meningococcemia infections, but can be seen in any patient with overwhelming infection.[35] Postsplenectomy sepsis syndrome patients and cancer patients are also at risk for purpura fulminans.[36] Patients present with signs of sepsis and the skin lesions often involve the extremities and may lead to amputation.

The best way to treat DIC is to treat the underlying cause (**Box 3**).[33] However, factors must be replaced if depletion occurs and bleeding ensues. Management should be guided using the five basic tests of coagulation (see **Box 2**).

Heparin therapy is reserved for the patient who has large vessel thrombosis as a component of their DIC.[37] Specific heparin levels should be used instead of the aPTT to monitor anticoagulation.[38] Cancer patients with chronic DIC will require long-term heparin therapy.

Box 3
Causes of DIC

Adenocarcinoma

Amniotic fluid embolism

Burns

Intravascular hemolysis

Infections

Leukemia

Penetrating brain injury

Placental abruption

Retained fetal death in utero

Shock

Snake bites

Trauma

PLATELET NUMBER AND FUNCTION
Immune Thrombocytopenia

Immune thrombocytopenia (ITP) is a common condition affecting about 1:20,000 individuals, most often young women. ITP most commonly complicates the care of patients with chronic lymphocytotic leukemia but can be seen with Hodgkin and non-Hodgkin lymphoma.[39] ITP is due to antibodies binding to platelet proteins, most often to the platelet receptor GP IIb/IIIa.[40] Patients often present with signs of bleeding and petechiae. Life-threatening bleeding is unusual and the physical examination is only remarkable for stigmata of bleeding such as petechiae. ITP can occur anytime in the course of the hematological neoplasm, ranging from predating the diagnosis to occurring when the patient is years in remission.

There is no specific laboratory test that "rules-in" ITP but rather it is a diagnosis of exclusion.[41] Extremely low platelet counts with a normal blood smear and a negative history can be diagnostic of ITP. The patient should be questioned carefully about drug exposure including over-the-counter medicines, natural remedies, or recreational drugs. Therapy in ITP should be guided by the patient's signs of bleeding and platelet counts. Overall, patients tolerate thrombocytopenia well. It is unusual to have life-threatening bleeding with platelet counts more than 1 to 5000/μL unless other sites of bleeding are present, such as a gastric ulcer. The primary therapy for ITP is pulse dexamethasone 40 mg/d for 4 days.[42] In patients with severe thrombocytopenia (counts less than 10,000/μL) or active bleeding, one of two treatments can be tried for rapid induction of a response. Either intravenous immune globulin at 1 g/kg repeated in 24 hours or intravenous anti-D antibody at 75 μg/kg single dose can induce a response in more than 80% of patients in 24 to 48 hours.[43,44]

Drug-induced Thrombocytopenia

Patients with drug-induced thrombocytopenia present with low platelet counts 1 to 3 weeks after starting a new medication.[45] In patients with a possible drug-induced thrombocytopenia, the primary therapy is to stop the suspect drug.[46] If there are multiple new medications, the best approach is to stop any drug that has been strongly associated with thrombocytopenia (**Box 4**). Immune globulin, corticosteroids, or intravenous anti—D have been suggested as useful in drug-related thrombocytopenia. However, because most of these thrombocytopenic patients recover when the agent is cleared from the body, this therapy is probably not necessary and avoids exposing the patients to the adverse events associated with further therapy.

Post-transfusion Purpura

In patients with post-transfusion purpura (PTP), the onset of severe thrombocytopenia (<10,000/μL), often with severe bleeding, will occur 1 to 2 weeks after receiving blood products.[47] These patients often lack platelet antigen PLA1. For unknown reasons, exposure to the antigens from the transfusion leads to rapid destruction of the patient's own platelets. The diagnostic clue is severe thrombocytopenia in a patient, typically female, who has received a red cell or platelet blood product in the past 7 to 10 days. Treatment consists of intravenous immunoglobulin[48] and plasmapheresis to remove the offending antibody. If patients with a history of PTP require further transfusions, only PLA1 negative platelets should be given.

Bleeding in the Platelet Refractory Patient

Many patients with cancer, particularly hematological cancers, become resistant to transfused platelets. Bleeding in patients who are refractory to platelet transfusion

---

Box 4
Common drugs implicated in thrombocytopenia

Anti-arrhythmic drugs
    Procainamide
    Quinidine
Anti GP IIb/IIIa agents
    Abciximab
    Eptifibatide
    Tirofiban
Antimicrobial
    Amphotericin B
    Rifampin
    Trimethoprim-sulfamethoxazole
    Vancomycin
H2-blockers
    Cimetidine
    Ranitidine
Acetaminophen
Amrirone
Carbamazepine
Efalizumab
Gold
Heparin
Hydrochlorothiazide
Nonsteroidal antiinflammatory agents
Quinine

---

presents a difficult clinical problem (**Box 5**).[49] If patients are shown to have HLA antibodies, HLA-matched platelets can be trnsfused.[50] Unfortunately, matched platelet transfusions may not be available and do not work in 20% to 70% of these patients. Even then, as many as 25% of patients have antiplatelet antibodies in which HLA-matched products will be ineffective. Platelet cross-matching can be performed to find compatible units for these patients, but this may not always be successful and may not be available in a timely manner. Use of antifibrinolytic agents such as ε-aminocaproic acid or tranexamic acid may decrease the incidence of bleeding. "Platelet drips" consisting of infusing either a platelet concentrate per hour or 1 plateletpheresis unit every 6 hours may be given as a continuous infusion. For life-threatening bleeding, rVIIa may be of use.[51] For platelet refractory patients with arterial bleeding, the use of angiographic delivery of platelets has been reported to be successful in stopping bleeding.[52]

Box 5
Emergency management of platelet alloimmunization

1. Evaluate for other causes of thrombocytopenia (heparin-induced thrombocytopenia [HIT], drugs).

2. Consider a platelet "drip" (1 unit of platelets given over 4–6 h).

3. Consider antifibrinolytic therapy:

   A. ε-Aminocaproic acid 1 g/h intravenously, or

   B. Tranexamic acid 10 mg/kg every 8 hours.

Heparin-induced Thrombocytopenia

Heparin-induced thrombocytopenia (HIT) occurs due to the formation of antibodies directed against the complex of heparin bonded to platelet factor 4, which results in a platelet and monocyte activation and thrombosis.[53] HIT is more common in cancer patients and has a higher rate of thrombotic complications.[54] The frequency of HIT is 1% to 5% if unfractionated heparin is used but less than 1% with low molecular weight heparin. HIT should be suspected if there is a sudden onset of thrombocytopenia with either at least a 50% drop in the platelet count from baseline or the platelet count falls to less than 100,000/μL in a patient receiving heparin in any form. HIT usually occurs 4 days after starting heparin but may occur suddenly in patients with recent (less than 3 months) exposure.[55–57] A feature of heparin-induced thrombocytopenia that is often overlooked is recurrent thrombosis in a patient receiving heparin despite a normal platelet count.[58] Patients with HIT can present to the ED up to 2 weeks after their hospital stay (and heparin exposure) with new thrombosis and thrombocytopenia.[59]

The diagnosis of HIT can be challenging in the cancer patient who has multiple reasons for being thrombocytopenic. In this situation, the laboratory assay for HIT may be helpful. Two general forms of HIT tests exist. One is a platelet aggregation assay whereby patient plasma, donor platelets, and heparin are added. If added heparin induces platelet aggregation, the test is considered positive. One caveat is that early in the HIT disease process the test can be negative but then turns positive 24 hours later as the antibody titer increases. There is also an ELISA assay for the presumed pathogenic antiplatelet factor 4 antibodies, which is sensitive but not specific. Positive ELISA results must be interpreted in the clinical context of the patient.

The first step in therapy for HIT consists of stopping all heparin. Low molecular weight heparins cross-react with the HIT antibodies and therefore these agents are also contraindicated.[55] Institution of warfarin therapy alone has been associated with an increased risk of thromboses.[55] For immediate antithrombotic therapy for HIT patients, three new antithrombotic agents are available (**Box 6**).[60,61] Patients with HIT should also be carefully screened for any thrombosis including examination by lower extremity Doppler ultrasound because of the propensity to have silent thrombosis.

Thrombotic Thrombocytopenic Purpura

Thrombotic thrombocytopenic purpura (TTP) should be suspected when a patient presents with any combination of thrombocytopenia, microangiopathic hemolytic anemia (schistocytes and signs of hemolysis), plus end-organ damage.[62] Patients

---

Box 6
Treatment of heparin-induced thrombocytopenia

Argatroban

Therapy: 2 μg/kg/min infusion with dose adjustments to keep aPTT 1.5 to 3 times normal. Decrease dose to 0.5 μg/kg/min in severe liver disease. For patients with multiorgan system failure, decrease dose to 1.0 μg/kg/min.

Lepirudin

Creatinine < 1.0 mg/dL: lepirudin starting infusion rate: 0.10 mg/kg/h

Creatinine, 1.0-1.6 mg/dL: starting infusion rate: 0.05 mg/kg/h;

Creatinine, 1.6-4.5 mg/dL: starting infusion rate: 0.01 mg/kg/h;

Creatinine > 4.5 mg/dL: starting infusion rate: 0.005 mg/kg/h)

- An initial intravenous bolus is no longer recommended unless there is life- or limb-threatening thrombosis; in these cases, the initial bolus dose is 0.2 mg/kg.

- aPTT performed at 4-h intervals until steady state within the therapeutic range (1.5- 2.0-times patient baseline aPTT) is achieved.

Fondaparinux

Prophylactic: 2.5 mg/d

Therapeutic: 7.5 mg/d (<50 kg, 5.0 mg/d; >100 kg, 10 mg/d)

---

with TTP most often present with intractable seizures, strokes, or sequela of renal insufficiency. Many patients who present with TTP have initially been misdiagnosed as having sepsis, lupus flare, or vasculitis.

There is currently no diagnostic test for TTP but rather the diagnosis is based on the clinical presentation.[63] Patients uniformly will have microangiopathic hemolytic anemia with the presence of schistocytes on the peripheral smear. Renal insufficiency and not frank renal failure is the most common renal manifestation. Thrombocytopenia may range from a minimal decrease in platelet number to an undetectable level of platelets. The lactate dehydrogenase (LDH) level is often elevated and is an important prognostic factor in TTP.[64] Untreated TTP is rapidly fatal. Mortality in the preplasma exchange era ranged from 95% to 100%. Today, plasma exchange therapy is the cornerstone of TTP treatment and has reduced mortality to less than 20%.[63,65,66]

Prednisone 1 mg/kg is routinely given to patents assumed to have TTP and should be continued until the patient has fully recovered. Although plasma infusion is beneficial, plasma exchange has been shown to be superior therapy for TTP.[65] This may be due to the large volumes of fresh frozen plasma and removal of inhibitory antibodies during plasma exchange. In patients who cannot be exchanged immediately, plasma infusions should be started at a dose of one unit every 4 hours. Patients with all but the mildest cases of TTP should receive 1.5 plasma volume exchange each day for at least 5 days.[63]

Therapy-related TTP/Hemolytic Uremic Syndrome

TTP/hemolytic uremic syndrome (HUS) can complicate a variety of therapies.[67] TTP/HUS can be associated with medications such as cyclosporine, FK506, mitomycin, and ticlopidine. With cyclosporine/FK506 the TTP/HUS occurs within days after the agent is started with the appearance of a falling platelet count, falling hematocrit, and rising serum LDH level.[68] Some cases have been fatal but often the TTP/HUS resolves after decreasing the dose of cyclosporine or changing to another agent.

TTP/HUS is most commonly seen with the antineoplastic agent mitomycin C with an incidence of 10% when a dose of more than 60 mg is used.[69] Anecdotal reports state that treatment with staphylococcal A columns may be useful for this condition.[70] Because advanced cancer itself can be associated with a TTP-like syndrome, the cause may be the underlying malignancy and not the cancer treatment.

TTP/HUS has been reported with other drugs including carboplatin, gemcitabine, and ticlopidine. The incidence of TTP with ticlopidine may be as high as 1:1600 and because this drug is often prescribed for patients with vascular disease, these patients may be initially misdiagnosed as having recurrent strokes or angina.[71] There are increasing reports of the antineoplastic agent gemcitabine causing TTP/HUS.[71] As with mitomycin, the appearance of the TTP/HUS syndrome with gemcitabine can be delayed and is often fatal. Severe hypertension often predates the clinical appearance of the TTP/HUS.[72]

TTP/HUS can complicate autologous and allogeneic bone marrow transplants.[73] The incidence ranges from 15% for allogeneic bone marrow transplants to 5% for autologous bone marrow transplants. Several types of TTP/HUS are recognized in bone marrow transplantation.[73,74] One is "multiorgan fulminant," which occurs early (20–60 days), has multiorgan system involvement, and is often fatal. Another type of TTP/HUS is similar to cyclosporin/FK506 HUS. A "conditioning" TTP/HUS, which occurs 6 months or more after total body irradiation, is associated with primary renal involvement. Finally, patients with systemic CMV infections can present with a TTP/HUS syndrome related to vascular infection with cytomegalovirus (CMV). The cause of bone marrow transplant–related TTP seems to be different from that of "classic" TTP because alterations of ADAMTS13 have not been found in bone marrow transplant–related TTP implicated in therapy-related vascular damage.[75] The therapy for bone marrow transplant TTP/HUS is uncertain. Patients should have their cyclosporine or FK506 doses decreased. Although plasma exchange is often tried, response is poor in fulminant- or conditioning-related TTP/HUS.[76]

Drug-Induced Hemolytic Disseminated Intravascular Coagulation Syndromes

A severe variant of the drug-induced immune complex hemolysis associated with DIC has been recognized. Patients who receive certain second and third generation cephalosporins (especially cefotetan and ceftriaxone) develop this syndrome, although this is rare.[77,78] The clinical syndrome starts 7 to 10 days after receiving the drug. Often the patient has only received the antibiotic for surgical prophylaxis. The patient will develop severe Coomb positive hemolysis with hypotension and DIC. The patients are often believed to have sepsis and are often re-exposed to cephalosporin, resulting in worsening of the clinical picture. The outcome is often fatal due to massive hemolysis and thrombosis.

Quinine is associated with a unique syndrome of drug-induced DIC.[79] Approximately 24 to 96 hours after exposure, the patient becomes acutely ill with nausea and vomiting. The patient then develops a microangiopathic hemolytic anemia, DIC, and renal failure. Some patients, besides having antiplatelet antibodies, also have antibodies binding to red cells and neutrophils that may lead to the more severe syndrome. Despite therapy, patients with quinine-induced TTP have a high incidence of chronic renal failure.

Treatment of drug-induced hemolytic DIC syndrome is anecdotal. Patients have responded to aggressive therapy including plasma exchange, dialysis, and prednisone.

Early recognition of the hemolytic anemia and the suspicion it is drug-related is important for early diagnosis so that the incriminating drug can be discontinued.

Uremia

Before the advent of dialysis, bleeding was a common late complication of uremia.[80] Bleeding in uremia is related to a platelet function defect; coagulation factors are not affected and unless other problems are present, the INR/aPTT are not prolonged.

The half-life of unfractionated and low molecular weight heparin is increased in renal failure.[81] Patients usually receive a bolus of heparin with dialysis and, rarely. patients will have a persistently prolonged anticoagulant effect. Low molecular weight heparins are cleared in the kidneys and if the dose is not adjusted, levels can greatly increase above therapeutic levels. Bleeding times are prolonged in renal disease, but there is little correlation between the bleeding time and clinical bleeding.[82]

Multiple treatment options exist for uremic bleeding including desmopressin, estrogen, and erythropoietin. Patients who are severely uremic and are bleeding may respond to aggressive dialysis.[83] Cryoprecipitate is not effective in some patients and its use exposes the patient to the risk of transfusion-transmitted viral disease.[84] Desmopressin is effective in uremic patients, with hemostasis being achieved for at least 4 to 8 hours after infusion.[85] Raising the hematocrit more than 30% by transfusions or erythropoietin will shorten the bleeding time in some situations.[86]

SPECIFIC HEMATOLOGICAL CANCERS ASSOCIATED WITH BLEEDING
Acute Promyelocytic Leukemia

The hemostatic defects in patients with acute promyelocytic leukemia (APL) are multiple.[87] Most if not all patients with APL have evidence of DIC at the time of diagnosis. Patients with APL have a higher risk of death during induction therapy compared with patients with other forms of leukemia, most often due to bleeding. Once in remission, patients with APL have a higher cure rate than most patients with leukemia. APL is also unique among leukemias in that biologic therapy with retinoic acid or arsenic is effective in inducing remission and cure in most patients.

APL patients can present with pancytopenia due to leukemic marrow replacement or with diffuse bleeding due to DIC and thrombocytopenia. Life-threatening bleeding such as intracranial hemorrhage may occur at any time until the leukemia is put into remission. The cause of the hemostatic defects in APL is complex and is believed to be the result of DIC, fibrinolysis, and the release of other procoagulant enzymes.[87] The diagnosis of APL can be straightforward when the leukemic cells are promyelocytes with abundant Auer rods, although some patients have the microgranular form without obvious Auer rods. The precise diagnosis requires molecular methods. On diagnosis of APL, a complete coagulation profile should be obtained including INR, aPTT, fibrinogen, platelet count, and D-dimer tests. Change in fibrinogen levels tends to be a good marker of progress in treating the coagulation defects.

Therapy for APL involves treating the leukemia and the coagulopathy. Currently the standard treatment of APL is *trans*-retinoic acid (ATRA) in combination with chemotherapy.[88] This will induce remission in more than 90% of patients, and a sizable number these patients will be cured of their APL. ATRA therapy will also lead to early correction of the coagulation defects, often within the first week of therapy, which is in stark contrast to the chemotherapy era when the coagulation defects would become worse with therapy.

Therapy for the coagulation defects consists of aggressive transfusion therapy support and possible use of other pharmacologic agents to control DIC.[89] One should try to maintain the fibrinogen level at more than 100 mg/dL and the platelet count at more than 50,000/μL. Controversy still exists over the role of heparin in therapy for APL.[90] Although attractive for its ability to neutralize thrombin, heparin use can lead to profound bleeding.

Other Leukemias and Myelodysplastic Syndromes

Along with the obvious thrombocytopenia due to marrow replacement, other coagulation defects may be seen in leukemias.[91] DIC can be seen in other forms of acute myelogenous leukemia apart from APL, such as acute monocytic leukemia. Patients with acute lymphocytic leukemia (ALL) may also have DIC often in association with induction therapy.

The most common coagulation defect in ALL is associated with the use of L-asparaginase.[92] Bleeding and thrombotic complications have been reported with the use of this effective chemotherapeutic agent. L-Asparaginase decreases hepatic synthesis of many proteins, including coagulation factors. Fortunately, despite low fibrinogen levels and markedly prolonged clotting times, bleeding is rarely seen. Paradoxically, thrombosis is seen in 0.5% to 4% of patients treated with L-asparaginase. These include strokes due to venous sinus or arterial thrombosis, as well as deep venous thrombosis and pulmonary embolism. Levels of the natural anticoagulants, such as protein S and antithrombin, are reduced with L-asparaginase and this may contribute to the hypercoagulable state. Patients with thrombosis should receive factor replacement and heparin.

Multiple defects are found in the platelets of patients with myelodysplastic syndrome. These include reduced platelet aggregation in response to a variety of agonists, decreased platelet stores of von Willebrand protein and fibrinogen. These patients may have severe bleeding even with platelet counts more than 50,000/μL. Platelet transfusion therapy for bleeding in myelodysplasia is often unsatisfactory.

Myeloproliferative Syndromes

A higher incidence of bleeding is seen in many of the myeloproliferative syndromes, but the bleeding rarely results in major morbidity.[89] A quarter of patients with polycythemia vera experience some bleeding but this is rarely the cause of death. Most series report that 30% of patients with essential thrombocytosis have bleeding. Paradoxically, the risk of bleeding seems to increase with platelet counts greater than 1 million. Some patients with extreme thrombocytosis have evidence of acquired von Willebrand disease.[24] Most bleeding in myeloproliferative syndromes consists of mucocutaneous bleeding or bruising with only a few reports of major bleeding. The use of drugs that inhibit platelet function is associated with a higher incidence of bleeding.

Therapy is nonspecific. Some patients with markedly elevated platelet counts will respond to lowering the counts to less than 1,000,000/μL.[24] This can be done rapidly by plateletpheresis or slowly (over days) by chemotherapy. Rarely, patients will have persistent oozing and bleeding after major procedures. Frequent platelet transfusions may be of value in these patients along with antifibrinolytic therapy.

Dysproteinemias

Dysproteinemia, the abnormal production of immunoglobulin, can affect many steps of the coagulation system and lead to severe bleeding. Multiple coagulation abnormalities have been described in patients with dysproteinemias.[93]

Therapy for the hemostatic defects in the dysproteinemic syndromes includes removal of the offending protein, either by reducing synthesis by treating the plasma cell dyscrasia or by intensive plasmapheresis. Patients with systemic amyloidosis, either primary or that associated with myeloma, often demonstrate a marked increase in easy bruising and other bleeding symptoms.[94] The most common defect in coagulation testing of patients with amyloidosis is an elevation in the thrombin time, which is seen in 30% to 80% of cases. An increased prothrombin time is seen in 20% to 24% of cases and an increased aPTT in up to 70%.

Another cause of bleeding in patients with systemic amyloidosis is systemic fibrinolysis. The mechanisms responsible for the fibrinolytic state are not known but hypotheses include increased release of plasminogen activators, decreased plasminogen activator inhibitors, blood vessels infiltrated with amyloid, decreased levels of inhibitors of fibrinolytic enzymes because of adsorption onto amyloid fibrils, or perhaps amyloid liver disease. The use of fibrinolytic inhibitors such as ε-aminocaproic acid or tranexamic acid has corrected fibrinolysis in laboratory tests and reduced bleeding symptoms.

COMPLICATIONS OF ANTITHROMBOTIC THERAPY
Antiplatelet Agents

For patients on aspirin with emergency bleeding, platelet transfusions can be given. The half-life of circulating aspirin is short, especially with low-dose therapy, and unless the patient has taken a dose within an hour of the transfusion the function of the transfused platelets should not be impaired. Desmopressin may reverse aspirin inhibition and is effective for emergency surgery in patients on aspirin therapy who are bleeding.[95] Little data exist on specific therapy for bleeding complications in patients using ticlopidine, clopidogrel, or prasugrel. All of these agents reduce the aggregation of platelets by irreversibly binding to $P2Y_{12}$ ADP receptors. For patients with severe bleeding, platelet transfusions may be used in an attempt to restore platelet function.

Therapy for bleeding complications associated with glycoprotein IIb/IIIa inhibitors is guided by the agent received. Most infused abciximab binds to the IIb/IIIa platelet receptor with little found free in the plasma.[96] Thus, for abciximab-related bleeding, treatment is to give a platelet transfusion, which will lead to redistribution of the abciximab over a wider number of receptors and return of platelet function. Tirofiban and eptifibatide do not bind as tightly so platelet transfusion may not fully restore platelet function. In vitro studies suggest that the addition of fibrinogen may help restore platelet function.[97] For severe bleeding, patients receiving tirofiban or eptifibatide should be transfused with 10 units of cryoprecipitate. Infusion of desmopressin 0.3 μg/kg may also be beneficial.[95]

Severe thrombocytopenia has been reported in 0.5% to 7.0% of patients receiving GP IIb/IIIa blockers,[98] higher in patients previously exposed.[99] All patients receiving these agents should have a platelet count checked 2 and 12 hours into therapy. The onset of the thrombocytopenia is rapid and can occur within 2 to 4 hours.[100] Experience with abciximab has shown that therapy with immune globulin or steroids is not helpful.

Warfarin

The key to management of an elevated INR is vitamin K (**Table 1**). Oral and intravenous vitamin K offer significant advantages over the use of subcutaneous vitamin K or plasma infusion. Often only small doses of vitamin K in the range of 0.5 to 3.0 mg are needed. Intravenous vitamin K, even if infused slowly, is associated with a slight risk of anaphylaxis (3:10,000).[101] For most situations, the oral route will result in reliable

Table 1
Management of high international normalized ratios

INR	Action
Not Bleeding: goal—INR back to therapeutic range in 24 h	
3–3.45	Hold dose until INR decreased
4.5–10	1 mg vitamin K by mouth
>10	2.5–5 mg vitamin K by mouth
Bleeding: goal—reversal of INR	
2–4.5	2.5 mg vitamin K + FFP
4.5–10	5 mg vitamin K + FFP
>10	5–10 mg vitamin K + FFP

Consider intravenous route for vitamin K if faster effect desired. For life-threatening bleeding give 10 mg vitamin K intravenously along with either rVIIa (40 μg/kg) or prothrombin complex concentrates (50 units/kg).

results, with an onset of action within 12 hours.[102] However, if speedy reversal is needed, then the intravenous route should be used because effects can be seen as soon as 4 hours.

For nonbleeding patients with high INRs less than five, vitamin K can simply be omitted or the dose lowered. There is a delay of 12 to 36 hours after stopping warfarin before the INR begins to decrease, so for INRs in the 5 to 10 range, the next 1 to 2 doses of warfarin should be held and 1.0 to 2.5 mg of vitamin K given orally. For INRs greater than 10, 2.5 to 5.0 mg of vitamin K should be given with the expectation that the INR will be lowered in 24 to 48 hours.

If the patient requires rapid full reversal because of bleeding or the need for surgery when the INR is 5 to 10, vitamin K can be given by the intravenous route[103] as well as fresh frozen plasma. Because one unit of plasma on average raises coagulation factors by only 5%, large doses (15 mg/kg or 4 to 5 units) must be given to attempt to completely correct the INR. As noted previously, transfusing this amount of plasma runs the risk of volume overload.

The rate of intracranial hemorrhage occurring in patients taking warfarin is 0.2% to 2%/year with the higher rates seen in older patients and with higher INRs.[104] These hemorrhages are particular devastating, with most patients either dying or incapacitated by the bleeding. Immediate management of bleeding is to rapidly reverse the warfarin effect.[105] This can be done by giving vitamin K (10 mg intravenous slowly over 1 hour) and fresh frozen plasma, or prothrombin complex concentrates (PCC). Clinical data have shown these products (which contain all the vitamin K-dependent clotting factors) result in a more rapid and complete correction of coagulation than plasma.[106] Patients suffering intracranial hemorrhages should receive PCC such as Konyne or Prophylnine at a dose of a 50 units/kg. Recent data also suggest that rVIIa is effective in reversing warfarin-induced bleeding.[105]

Heparin

Standard heparin has a short (30–60 minutes) half-life, so in most situations reversal is not required. Low molecular weight heparins have a half-life of several hours, so reversal may be required for serious bleeding soon after drug administration. Protamine is used to reverse heparin and low molecular weight heparin. The dose for heparin reversal is dependent on the timing of the last heparin dose. For immediate reversal (30 minutes or less since the last heparin dose), 1 mg of protamine should be given for every 100 units of heparin. For 30 to 60 minutes after the dose, 0.5 mg of protamine for every 100 units of heparin should be given, and for 60 to 120 minutes, 0.375 mg of protamine for every 100 units of heparin.[107] The infusion rate of protamine should not exceed 5 mg/min.[107]

Protamine does not fully reverse low molecular weight heparin but can neutralize the antithrombin effect.[108] Due to the longer half-life of low molecular weight heparin, sometimes a second dose of protamine is required. The dose is 1 mg/100 units of daltaparin or tinzaparin or 1 mg/mg of enoxaparin. If the aPTT is prolonged, 4 hours later (reflecting continued thrombin inhibition), one half of the initial dose should be given.

New Agents

Currently no effective antidote exists for fondaparinux or the newer oral agents such as the Xa blockers rivaroxaban, apixiban, and the direct thrombin inhibitor dibigatran.[109] There are data that rVIIa may reverse the coagulation defect in vitro but the clinical usefulness of this is unknown.[110] The half-lives of the oral agents are relative short (4–8 hours) so the drug effect will dissipate quickly except for fondaparinux whose half-life is 18 to 21 hours.

Fibrinolytic Agents

The major complication of thrombolytic therapy is bleeding. Rates of major bleeding range from 4.6% to 5.94%.[96] Patients bleed at sites of previous injury due to lysis of previously formed thrombosis or due to underlying vascular problems such as cerebral vascular amyloid.[111] The most devastating complication is intracerebral hemorrhage (ICH), which can have a mortality rate of up to 60%.[112] ICH occurs in approximately 0.4% to 0.8% of patients with acute myocardial infarction[113] and 1% to 2% of patients with pulmonary embolism or deep venous thrombosis.[114] The highest rates of ICH are seen in patients receiving thrombolytic therapy for stroke with rates of 3% to 15%.[115] Older patients (>75 years), smaller patients, patients with previous stoke, hypertensive patients, and those receiving tPA are at higher risk of bleeding.[116] Patients will have a low fibrinogen level, elevated INR and aPTT due to destruction of factors V and VIII, and abnormal platelet function and lysis of formed thrombi. Patients who suffer severe bleeding after thrombolytic therapy[117] should be infused with cryoprecipitate to replace fibrinogen as well as factor VIII and platelets. If the patient is having an intracranial hemorrhage, empirical therapy with cryoprecipitate, platelets, and plasma should be given. Although reversal of the fibrinolytic state can be achieved with the use of antifibrinolytic agents, this is rarely required, as the fibrinolytic state, especially with tPA, is short-lived.

SUMMARY

Numerous factors can lead to bleeding in cancer patients. Many of these can be deduced from a good history – knowing the cancer diagnosis, type of therapy received, assessing if the patient is on anticoagulants – and reviewing basic hemostatic tests. Management of severe bleeding is guided by these basic tests and transfusion of blood products. DIC can be a primary complication of cancer or a sequela of sepsis due to immunosuppression. Specific cancers – especially hematological neoplasms – can induce bleeding disorders. Finally, given the propensity of cancer patients to have thrombosis, bleeding from antithrombotic therapy is always a threat.

REFERENCES

1. Biron C, Bengler C, Gris JC, et al. Acquired isolated factor VII deficiency during sepsis. Haemostasis 1997;27(2):51–6.
2. Peterson P, Hayes TE, Arkin CF, et al. The preoperative bleeding time test lacks clinical benefit: College of American Pathologists' and American Society of Clinical Pathologists' position article. Arch Surg 1998;133(2):134–9.
3. Ortel TL, James AH, Thames EH, et al. Assessment of primary hemostasis by PFA-100 analysis in a tertiary care center. Thromb Haemost 2000;84(1):93–7.
4. Whitten CW, Greilich PE. Thromboelastography: past, present, and future. Anesthesiology 2000;92(5):1223–5.
5. Wilson RF, Mammen E, Walt AJ. Eight years of experience with massive blood transfusions. J Trauma 1971;11(4):275–85.
6. Hébert PC, Wells G, Blajchman MA, et al. A multicenter, randomized, controlled clinical trial of transfusion requirements in critical care. N Engl J Med 1999; 340(6):409–17.
7. Counts RB, Haisch C, Simon TL, et al. Hemostasis in massively transfused trauma patients. Ann Surg 1979;190(1):91–9.
8. Chowdhury P, Saayman AG, Paulus U, et al. Efficacy of standard dose and 30 ml/kg fresh frozen plasma in correcting laboratory parameters of haemostasis in critically ill patients. Br J Haematol 2004;125(1):69–73.
9. Hirshberg A, Dugas M, Banez EI, et al. Minimizing dilutional coagulopathy in exsanguinating hemorrhage: a computer simulation. J Trauma 2003;54(3):454–63.
10. Sperry JL, Ochoa JB, Gunn SR, et al. An FFP: PRBC transfusion ratio >/=1:1.5 is associated with a lower risk of mortality after massive transfusion. J Trauma 2008;65(5):986–93.
11. Tisherman SA. Hypothermia and injury. Curr Opin Crit Care 2004;10(6):512–9.
12. Rajek A, Greif R, Sessler DI, et al. Core cooling by central venous infusion of ice-cold (4 degrees C and 20 degrees C) fluid: isolation of core and peripheral thermal compartments. Anesthesiology 2000;93(3):629–37.
13. Howland WS, Schwiezer O, Boyan CP. Massive blood replacement without calcium administration. Surg Gynecol Obstet 1964;159:171–7.
14. Miller RD, Tong MJ, Robbins TO. Effects of massive transfusion of blood on acid-base balance. JAMA 1971;216(11):1762–5.
15. Hay CR, Negrier C, Ludlam CA. The treatment of bleeding in acquired haemophilia with recombinant factor VIIa: a multicentre study. Thromb Haemost 1997; 78(6):1463–7.
16. DeLoughery TG. Management of bleeding emergencies: when to use recombinant activated factor VII. Expert Opin Pharmacother 2006;7(1):25–34.
17. Birchall J, Stanworth SJ, Duffy MR, et al. Evidence for the use of recombinant factor VIIa in the prevention and treatment of bleeding in patients without hemophilia. Transfus Med Rev 2008;22(3):177–87.
18. Dutton RP, Hess JR, Scalea TM. Recombinant factor VIIa for control of hemorrhage: early experience in critically ill trauma patients. J Clin Anesth 2003; 15(3):184–8.
19. Martinowitz U, Michaelson M. Guidelines for the use of recombinant activated factor VII (rFVIIa) in uncontrolled bleeding: a report by the Israeli Multidisciplinary rFVIIa task force. J Thromb Haemost 2005;3:640–8.
20. Abshire T, Kenet G. Recombinant factor VIIa: review of efficacy, dosing regimens and safety in patients with congenital and acquired factor VII or IX inhibitors. J Thromb Haemost 2004;2:899–909.

21. Pavese P, Bonadona A, Beaubien J, et al. FVIIa corrects the coagulopathy of fulminant hepatic failure but may be associated with thrombosis: a report of four cases. Can J Anaesth 2005;52(1):26–9.

22. Mayer SA, Brun NC, Begtrup K, et al. Efficacy and safety of recombinant activated factor VII for acute intracerebral hemorrhage. N Engl J Med 2008; 358(20):2127–37.

23. Tefferi A, Nichols WL. Acquired von Willebrand disease: concise review of occurrence, diagnosis, pathogenesis, and treatment. Am J Med 1997;103(6): 536–40.

24. Eikenboom JC, Tjernberg P, Van M, et al. Acquired von Willebrand syndrome: diagnostic problems and therapeutic options. Am J Hematol 2007;82(1):55–8.

25. Michiels JJ, Budde U, van der PM, et al. Acquired von Willebrand syndromes: clinical features, aetiology, pathophysiology, classification and management. Best Pract Res Clin Haematol 2001;14(2):401–36.

26. Facon T, Caron C, Courtin P, et al. Acquired type II von Willebrand's disease associated with adrenal cortical carcinoma. Br J Haematol 1992;80:488–94.

27. van Genderen PJ, Michiels JJ. Acquired von Willebrand disease. Baillieres Clin Haematol 1998;11(2):319–30.

28. Federici AR. Therapeutic approaches to acquired von Willebrand syndrome. Expert Opin Investig Drugs 2000;9(2):347–54.

29. Federici AB, Stabile F, Castaman G, et al. Treatment of acquired von Willebrand syndrome in patients with monoclonal gammopathy of uncertain significance: comparison of three different therapeutic approaches. Blood 1998;92(8): 2707–11.

30. Friederich PW, Wever PC, Briet E, et al. Successful treatment with recombinant factor VIIa of therapy-resistant severe bleeding in a patient with acquired von Willebrand disease. Am J Hematol 2001;66:292–4.

31. Franchini M, Lippi G. Acquired factor VIII inhibitors. Blood 2008;112(2):250–5.

32. Barnett B, Kruse-Jarres R, Leissinger CA. Current management of acquired factor VIII inhibitors. Curr Opin Hematol 2008;15(5):451–5.

33. Levi M, ten Cate H. Disseminated intravascular coagulation. N Engl J Med 1999; 341(8):586–92.

34. Davis MD, Dy KM, Nelson S. Presentation and outcome of purpura fulminans associated with peripheral gangrene in 12 patients at Mayo Clinic. J Am Acad Dermatol 2007;57(6):944–56.

35. Gamper G, Oschatz E, Herkner H, et al. Sepsis-associated purpura fulminans in adults. Wien Klin Wochenschr 2001;113(3–4):107–12.

36. Carpenter CT, Kaiser AB. Purpura fulminans in pneumococcal sepsis: case report and review. Scand J Infect Dis 1997;29(5):479–83.

37. Feinstein DI. Diagnosis and management of disseminated intravascular coagulation: the role of heparin therapy. Blood 1982;60(2):284–7.

38. Olson JD, Arkin CF, Brandt JT, et al. College of American Pathologists Conference XXXI on laboratory monitoring of anticoagulant therapy: laboratory monitoring of unfractionated heparin therapy. Arch Pathol Lab Med 1998;122(9): 782–98.

39. Ding W, Zent CS. Diagnosis and management of autoimmune complications of chronic lymphocytic leukemia/small lymphocytic lymphoma. Clin Adv Hematol Oncol 2007;5(4):257–61.

40. McMillan R, Lopez-Dee J, Bowditch R. Clonal restriction of platelet-associated anti-GPIIb/IIIa autoantibodies in patients with chronic ITP. Thromb Haemost 2001;85(5):821–3.

41. Godeau B, Provan D, Bussel J. Immune thrombocytopenic purpura in adults. Curr Opin Hematol 2007;14(5):535–56.
42. Mazzucconi MG, Fazi P, Bernasconi S, et al. Therapy with high-dose dexamethasone (HD-DXM) in previously untreated patients affected by idiopathic thrombocytopenic purpura: a GIMEMA experience. Blood 2007;109(4): 1401–7.
43. Newman GC, Novoa MV, Fodero EM, et al. A dose of 75 microg/kg/d of i.v. anti-D increases the platelet count more rapidly and for a longer period of time than 50 microg/kg/d in adults with immune thrombocytopenic purpura. Br J Haematol 2001;112(4):1076–8.
44. Lazarus AH, Freedman J, Semple JW. Intravenous immunoglobulin and anti-D in idiopathic thrombocytopenic purpura (ITP): mechanisms of action. Transfus Sci 1998;19(3):289–94.
45. Aster RH, Bougie DW. Drug-induced immune thrombocytopenia. N Engl J Med 2007;357(6):580–7.
46. Zondor SD, George JN, Medina PJ. Treatment of drug-induced thrombocytopenia. Expert Opin Drug Saf 2002;1(2):173–80.
47. Mueller-Eckhardt C. Post-transfusion purpura. Br J Haematol 1986;64(3): 419–24.
48. Mueller-Eckhardt C, Kiefel V. High-dose IgG for post-transfusion purpura-revisited. Blut 1988;57(4):163–7.
49. Dan ME, Schiffer CA. Strategies for managing refractoriness to platelet transfusions. Curr Hematol Rep 2003;2(2):158–64.
50. Schiffer CA. Diagnosis and management of refractoriness to platelet transfusion. Blood Rev 2001;15(4):175–80.
51. Kirkpatrick BD, Alston WK. Current immunizations for travel. Curr Opin Infect Dis 2003;16(5):369–74.
52. Madoff DC, Wallace MJ, Lichtiger B, et al. Intraarterial platelet infusion for patients with intractable gastrointestinal hemorrhage and severe refractory thrombocytopenia. J Vasc Interv Radiol 2004;15(4):393–7.
53. Warkentin TE. Heparin-induced thrombocytopenia. Hematol Oncol Clin North Am 2007;21(4):589–607, v.
54. Opatrny L, Warner MN. Risk of thrombosis in patients with malignancy and heparin-induced thrombocytopenia. Am J Hematol 2004;76(3):240–4.
55. Warkentin TE. Heparin-induced thrombocytopenia: a ten-year retrospective. Annu Rev Med 1999;50:129–47.
56. Srichaikul T, Nimmannitya S. Haematology in denque and denque haemorrhagic fever. Baillieres Clin Haematol 2000;13:261–76.
57. Cvachovec K, Horacek M, Vislocky I. A retrospective survey of fibrinolysis as an indicator of poor outcome after cardiopulmonary bypass and a possible early sign of systemic inflammation syndrome. Eur J Anaesthesiol 2000; 17(3):173–6.
58. Hach-Wunderle V, Kainer K, Krug B, et al. Heparin-associated thrombosis despite normal platelet counts. Lancet 1994;344:469–70.
59. Smythe MA, Stephens JL, Mattson JC. Delayed-onset heparin-induced thrombocytopenia. Ann Emerg Med 2005;45(4):417–9.
60. Laposata M, Green D, Van Cott EM, et al. College of American Pathologists Conference XXXI on Laboratory Monitoring of Anticoagulant Therapy - the clinical use and laboratory monitoring of low-molecular-weight heparin, danaparoid, hirudin and related compounds, and argatroban. Arch Pathol Lab Med 1998; 122:799–807.

61. Hirsh J, Warkentin TE, Raschke R, et al. Heparin and low-molecular-weight heparin - mechanisms of action, pharmacokinetics, dosing considerations, monitoring, efficacy, and safety. Chest 1998;114(Suppl):489S–510S.

62. Murrin RJ, Murray JA. Thrombotic thrombocytopenic purpura: aetiology, pathophysiology and treatment. Blood Rev 2006;20(1):51–60.

63. George JN. How I treat patients with thrombotic thrombocytopenic purpura-hemolytic uremic syndrome. Blood 2000;96:1223–9.

64. Patton JF, Manning KR, Case D, et al. Serum lactate dehydrogenase and platelet count predict survival in thrombotic thrombocytopenic purpura. Am J Hematol 1994;47:94–9.

65. Rock GA, Shumak KH, Buskard NA, et al. Comparison of plasma exchange with plasma infusion in the treatment of thrombotic thrombocytopenic purpura. N Engl J Med 1991;325:393–7.

66. Bell WR, Braine HG, Ness PM, et al. Improved survival in thrombotic thrombocytopenic purpura- hemolytic uremic syndrome – clinical experience in 108 patients. N Engl J Med 1991;325:398–403.

67. Moake JL, Byrnes JJ. Thrombotic microangiopathies associated with drugs and bone marrow transplantation. Hematol Oncol Clin North Am 1996;10(2):485–97.

68. Gharpure VS, Devine SM, Holland HK, et al. Thrombotic thrombocytopenic purpura associated with FK506 following bone marrow transplantation. Bone Marrow Transplant 1995;16(5):715–6.

69. Wu DC, Liu JM, Chen YM, et al. Mitomycin-C induced hemolytic uremic syndrome: a case report and literature review. Jpn J Clin Oncol 1997;27(2): 115–8.

70. Borghardt EJ, Kirchertz EJ, Marten I, et al. Protein A-immunoadsorption in chemotherapy associated hemolytic-uremic syndrome. Transfus Sci 1998; 19(Suppl):5–7.

71. Saif MW, McGee PJ. Hemolytic-uremic syndrome associated with gemcitabine: a case report and review of literature. JOP 2005;6(4):369–74.

72. Walter RB, Joerger M, Pestalozzi BC. Gemcitabine-associated hemolytic-uremic syndrome. Am J Kidney Dis 2002;40(4):E16.

73. Clark RE. Thrombotic microangiopathy following bone marrow transplantation [see comments]. Bone Marrow Transplant 1994;14(4):495–504.

74. Fuge R, Bird JM, Fraser A, et al. The clinical features, risk factors and outcome of thrombotic thrombocytopenic purpura occurring after bone marrow transplantation. Br J Haematol 2001;113(1):58–64.

75. Van der Plas RM, Schiphorst ME, Huizinga EG, et al. von Willebrand factor proteolysis is deficient in classic, but not in bone marrow transplantation-associated, thrombotic thrombocytopenic purpura. Blood 1999;93(11):3798–802.

76. Sarode R, McFarland JG, Flomenberg N, et al. Therapeutic plasma exchange does not appear to be effective in the management of thrombotic thrombocytopenic purpura/hemolytic uremic syndrome following bone marrow transplantation. Bone Marrow Transplant 1995;16(2):271–5.

77. Garratty G. Immune cytopenia associated with antibiotics. Transfus Med Rev 1993;7(4):255–67.

78. Seltsam A, Salama A. Ceftriaxone-induced immune haemolysis: two case reports and a concise review of the literature. Intensive Care Med 2000;26(9): 1390–4.

79. Kojouri K, Vesely K, George JN. Quinine-induced thrombotic thrombocytopenic purpura - hemolytic uremic syndrome (TTP-HUS): frequency, clinical features, and long-term outcomes. Ann Intern Med 2001;135(12):1047–51.

80. Escolar G, Díaz-Ricart M, Cases A. Uremic platelet dysfunction: past and present. Curr Hematol Rep 2005;4(5):359–67.
81. Chow SL, Zammit K, West K, et al. Correlation of antifactor Xa concentrations with renal function in patients on enoxaparin. J Clin Pharmacol 2003;43(6):586–90.
82. Rodgers RP, Levin J. A critical reappraisal of the bleeding time. Semin Thromb Hemost 1990;16(1):1–20.
83. Andrassy K, Ritz E. Uremia as a cause of bleeding. Am J Nephrol 1985;5(5): 313–9.
84. Triulzi DJ, Blumberg N. Variability in response to cryoprecipitate treatment for hemostatic defects in uremia. Yale J Biol Med 1990;63(1):1–7.
85. Weigert AL, Schafer AI. Uremic bleeding: pathogenesis and therapy. Am J Med Sci 1998;316(2):94–104.
86. Moia M, Mannucci PM, Vizzotto L, et al. Improvement in the haemostatic defect of uraemia after treatment with recombinant human erythropoietin. Lancet 1987; 2(8570):1227–9.
87. Arbuthnot C, Wilde JT. Haemostatic problems in acute promyelocytic leukaemia. Blood Rev 2006;20(6):289–97.
88. Wang ZY, Chen Z. Acute promyelocytic leukemia: from highly fatal to highly curable. Blood 2008;111(5):2505–15.
89. Falanga A, Rickles FR. Management of thrombohemorrhagic syndromes (THS) in hematologic malignancies. Hematology Am Soc Hematol Educ Program 2007;2007:165–71.
90. Sanz MA, Grimwade D, Tallman MS, et al. Guidelines on the management of acute promyelocytic leukemia: recommendations from an expert panel on behalf of the European LeukemiaNet. Blood 2009;113(9):1875–91.
91. Uchiumi H, Matsushima T, Yamane A, et al. Prevalence and clinical characteristics of acute myeloid leukemia associated with disseminated intravascular coagulation. Int J Hematol 2007;86(2):137–42.
92. DeLoughery TG, Goodnight SH, et al. Bleeding and thrombosis in hematologic neoplasia. In: Wiernik PH, Canellos GP, Dutcher JP, editors. Neoplastic diseases of the blood. 3rd edition. New York: Churchill Livingston; 1996. p. 1177–92.
93. Zangari M, Elice F, Fink L, et al. Hemostatic dysfunction in paraproteinemias and amyloidosis. Semin Thromb Hemost 2007;33(4):339–49.
94. Eby CS. Bleeding and thrombosis risks in plasma cell dyscrasias. Hematology Am Soc Hematol Educ Program 2007;2007:158–64.
95. Reiter RA, Mayr F, Blazicek H, et al. Desmopressin antagonizes the in vitro platelet dysfunction induced by GPIIb/IIIa inhibitors and aspirin. Blood 2003; 102(13):4594–9.
96. Schroeder WS, Gandhi PJ. Emergency management of hemorrhagic complications in the era of glycoprotein IIb/IIIa receptor antagonists, clopidogrel, low molecular weight heparin, and third-generation fibrinolytic agents. Curr Cardiol Rep 2003;5(4):310–7.
97. Li YF, Spencer FA, Becker RC. Comparative efficacy of fibrinogen and platelet supplementation on the in vitro reversibility of competitive glycoprotein IIb/IIIa receptor-directed platelet inhibition. Am Heart J 2002;143(4):725–32.
98. Berkowitz SD, Sane DC, Sigmon KN, et al. Occurrence and clinical significance of thrombocytopenia in a population undergoing high-risk percutaneous coronary revascularization. J Am Coll Cardiol 1998;32:311–9.
99. Ibbotson T, McGavin JK, Goa KL. Abciximab: an updated review of its therapeutic use in patients with ischaemic heart disease undergoing percutaneous coronary revascularisation. Drugs 2003;63(11):1121–63.

100. Berkowitz SD, Harrington RA, Rund MM, et al. Acute profound thrombocytopenia after c7E3 Fab (abciximab) therapy. Circulation 1997;95:809–13.

101. Riegert-Johnson DL, Volcheck GW. The incidence of anaphylaxis following intravenous phytonadione (vitamin K1): a 5-year retrospective review. Ann Allergy Asthma Immunol 2002;89(4):400–6.

102. Whitling AM, Bussey HI, Lyons RM. Comparing different routes and doses of phytonadione for reversing excessive anticoagulation. Arch Intern Med 1998; 158(19):2136–40.

103. Makris M, Watson HG. The management of coumarin-induced over-anticoagulation annotation. Br J Haematol 2001;114(2):271–80.

104. Schulman S, Beyth RJ, Kearon C, et al. Hemorrhagic complications of anticoagulant and thrombolytic treatment: American College of Chest Physicians Evidence-Based Clinical Practice Guidelines. (8th edition). Chest 2008;133(6 Suppl):257S–98S.

105. Aguilar MI, Hart RG, Kase CS, et al. Treatment of warfarin-associated intracerebral hemorrhage: literature review and expert opinion. Mayo Clin Proc 2007; 82(1):82–92.

106. Leissinger CA, Blatt PM, Hoots WK, et al. Role of prothrombin complex concentrates in reversing warfarin anticoagulation: a review of the literature. Am J Hematol 2008;83(2):137–43.

107. Monagle P, Michelson AD, Bovill E, et al. Antithrombotic therapy in children. Chest 2001;119(1 Suppl):344S–70S.

108. Holst J, Lindblad B, Bergqvist D, et al. Protamine neutralization of intravenous and subcutaneous low-molecular-weight heparin (tinzaparin, logiparin). An experimental investigation in healthy volunteers. Blood Coagul Fibrinolysis 1994;5(5):795–803.

109. Weitz JI. Emerging anticoagulants for the treatment of venous thromboembolism. Thromb Haemost 2006;96(3):274–84.

110. Lisman T, Bijsterveld NR, Adelmeijer J, et al. Recombinant factor VIIa reverses the in vitro and ex vivo anticoagulant and profibrinolytic effects of fondaparinux. J Thromb Haemost 2003;1(11):2368–73.

111. Sloan MA, Price TR, Petito CK, et al. Clinical features and pathogenesis of intracerebral hemorrhage after rt-PA and heparin therapy for acute myocardial infarction: the Thrombolysis in Myocardial Infarction (TIMI) II pilot and randomized clinical trial combined experience. Neurology 1995;45:649–58.

112. Sloan MA, Sila CA, Mahaffey KW, et al. Prediction of 30-day mortality among patients with thrombolysis-related intracranial hemorrhage. Circulation 1998; 98(14):1376–82.

113. Brass LM, Lichtman JH, Wang Y, et al. Intracranial hemorrhage associated with thrombolytic therapy for elderly patients with acute myocardial infarction: results from the cooperative cardiovascular project. Stroke 2000;31(8):1802–11.

114. Patel SC, Mody A. Cerebral hemorrhagic complications of thrombolytic therapy. Prog Cardiovasc Dis 1999;42(3):217–33.

115. Graham GD. Tissue plasminogen activator for acute ischemic stroke in clinical practice: a meta-analysis of safety data. Stroke 2003;34(12):2847–50.

116. Mehta SR, Eikelboom JW, Yusuf S. Risk of intracranial haemorrhage with bolus versus infusion thrombolytic therapy: a meta-analysis. [comment] Lancet 2000; 356(9228):449–54.

117. Sane DC, Califf RM, Topol EJ, et al. Bleeding during thrombolytic therapy for acute myocardial infarction: mechanism and management. Ann Intern Med 1989;111:1010–22.

Radiation Therapy– Related Toxicity (Including Pneumonitis and Fibrosis)

Rahul R. Chopra, MD*, Jeffrey A. Bogart, MD

KEYWORDS

- Radiation therapy • Toxicity • Inflammation
- Corticosteroids • Endarteritis • Fibrosis

In the modern age of cancer therapy, multidisciplinary management has led to increasing rates of survivorship. Surgery, chemotherapy, and radiation therapy (RT) are often integrated to optimize the likelihood of local control and survival for a wide spectrum of malignancies. RT toxicity must be tempered with the desire to deliver intensive therapy with the goal of improving tumor control and cure. The differential diagnosis for many RT-related toxicities is extensive. Several factors can modulate RT-related toxicity, including ancillary treatments, such as surgery and chemotherapy, as well as the underlying nutritional and medical status of the patient. This article is designed to acquaint emergency medicine physicians with common toxic effects in patients undergoing RT.

THERAPEUTIC MECHANISM OF CLINICAL RADIATION THERAPY

The principal therapeutic beam in radiation oncology is the x-ray (or γ-ray), and it consists of a large number of photons, or "packets," of energy.[1] The absorption of energy from radiation in a biologic material may lead to excitation or to ionization within the atoms of the biologic tissue.[2] The raising of an electron in an atom or molecule to a higher energy level without actual ejection of the electron is called excitation. If the photon is of sufficient energy, ejection of 1 or more orbital electrons from the atom can occur, and this process is referred to as ionization. The radiation that causes this is referred to as ionizing radiation.[2] The most important characteristic of ionizing radiation is the localized release of large amounts of energy. The energy dissipated per

A version of this article was previously published in the *Emergency Medicine Clinics of North America*, 27:2.

Department of Radiation Oncology, State University of New York Upstate Medical University, 750 East Adams Street, Syracuse, NY 13210, USA

* Corresponding author.

E-mail address: choprar@upstate.edu

ionizing event (33 eV) is more than enough to break strong chemical bonds. Charged particles, such as electrons, protons, and α-particles, are *directly* ionizing, whereas uncharged particles, such as photons and neutrons, are *indirectly* ionizing.[1] Provided that charged particles have sufficient kinetic energy, they can directly disrupt the atomic structure of the biologic material through which they pass, creating chemical and biologic damage. Uncharged particles, with energy similar to photons, do not directly produce chemical and biologic damage themselves, but when they are absorbed in the material through which they pass, they give up their energy to produce fast-moving charged particles, known as free radicals, that are able to produce damage.

Conventional RT involves using x-rays to produce biologic damage. When a photon hits a water molecule in a cell, generation of a hydroxyl free radical occurs. It is estimated that two-thirds of the x-ray damage to DNA in mammalian cells is caused by the hydroxyl radical.[2] Damage to cellular DNA is the primary mechanism through which radiation is able to exert its therapeutic effect. When a cancer attempts to divide with a damaged genome, it undergoes a mitotic death.

RADIOBIOLOGICAL EFFECTS OF RADIATION THERAPY AT THE CELLULAR AND TISSUE LEVEL

RT is a local modality that generally causes toxicity limited to the area of treatment (with some caveats). The effects of RT on normal tissues generally result from the depletion of a cell population by cell killing. The cells of normal tissue are not independent units but rather form a complete integrated structure. Response to RT is governed by 3 main factors: (1) inherent cellular radiosensitivity, (2) kinetics of the tissue, and (3) organization of cells within the tissue. Visible damage to an organ becomes evident only if a sufficient proportion of cells are killed. As mentioned previously, cell death after irradiation occurs when cells try to divide. In tissues with rapid turnover, damage can become evident quickly—in a matter of hours (as in gastrointestinal [GI] mucosa) or days (skin). This gives rise to the concept of "early" responding tissues. "Late" responding tissues have toxicity that occurs after a delay of months or years and predominantly in slowly proliferating tissues, such as the lung, kidney, heart, liver, and the central nervous system (CNS).[3] Acute damage is generally repaired quickly secondary to rapid proliferation of underlying stem cells. Late effects, in contrast, may improve but never completely repair. A late effect generally results from a combination of vascular damage through radiation endarteritis in combination with a loss of parenchymal cells. Radiation endarteritis leads to significant atherosclerotic disease several years after initial therapy, in the areas that previously received RT. If an intensive radiation regimen is used with subsequent depletion of the stem-cell population below levels needed for tissue repair, an early reaction in a rapidly proliferating tissue may persist as a chronic injury. This is termed a consequential late effect.[3] An example of this would be necrosis or fibrosis of the skin that occur consequent to severe radiation dermatitis and acute ulceration.

Another concept that is important in understanding radiation toxicity is the idea of an underlying organ's makeup, namely its functional subunits. The tolerance of normal tissues to radiation is dependent on the ability of clonogenic tissue progenitor cells to maintain a sufficient number of differentiated cells that are appropriately structured to maintain organ function. The structural organization of a tissue is crucial in determining the relationship between survival of clonogenic progenitor cells and organ function versus failure. Structurally *defined* functional subunits can include the hepatic lobule, the renal nephron, or the pulmonary acinus. Structurally *undefined* functional units are seen in the cutaneous skin where re-epithelialization of a denuded area can occur either from surviving clonogens within the affected area or by migration from adjacent areas. In the case of organs such as the lung, liver, and kidney, a certain portion can be treated without significant dysfunction. The subunits in these tissues work in *parallel* to carry out the physiologic function. This is in contrast to *serial* tissues, such as the spinal cord, where disruption of a portion of the tissue affects all downstream activity.[3]

RT is generally given as a number of small doses on a daily basis, rather than one large fraction (although this does occur as well and is generally referred to as radiosurgery). Dividing a dose into a number of smaller doses, or fractions, allows normal tissues to be spared. This is due to repair of cellular damage that occurs each day. Normal cells typically have better repair mechanisms than those of cancer cells, and RT is used to exploit this difference. Prolonging overall treatment time and decreasing fraction size will generally decrease the severity of "early" effects. Increasing the dose of radiation per fraction to normal tissue may not affect the patient acutely but results in an increased risk of "late" effects several months to several years later.[3] A review of classically defined radiation tolerance is shown in **Table 1**. The TD 5/5 and TD 50/5 in **Table 1** refer to radiation doses that would be expected to cause a 5% or 50% rate of the given complication or toxicity at 5 years.

TOXICITY BY ORGAN SYSTEM
Skin and Soft Tissue Toxicity

Acute radiation toxicity of the skin generally has a time course of several days to weeks after beginning RT. Before the advent of modern megavoltage linear accelerators, acute skin toxicity was the most common dose-limiting factor. Clinical signs of acute radiation toxicity can include erythema, edema, and hyperpigmentation. At higher doses, both moist desquamation and dry desquamation can occur.[4] Management generally consists of cleansers, moisturizers, petrolatum-based products (for dry desquamation), topical steroids (somewhat controversial), wound cleaners/epithelial stimulants, and hydrocolloid dressings.[5] Skin reactions are typically self-limited and will resolve over a matter of a few weeks' time. In some cases with severe desquamation, topical burn medication such as silvadene cream may be required, and patients may need to be admitted for wound management and antibiotics for a potential superinfection.

Fibrosis is one of the most common chronic skin and soft tissue toxicities that occur in patients who have undergone RT, with a time course that begins several months to a few years after completing RT. This may occur in the absence of a severe acute skin reaction. The etiology is thought to be a characteristic RT-induced endarteritis with vascular and capillary damage. Chronic tissue hypoxia leads to fibroblast proliferation and eventual scarring and fibrosis of the affected tissue. As with any late effect, dose, volume, and RT fractionation can affect the eventual clinical outcome. Other factors such as previous surgical manipulation and underlying medical comorbidities, such as diabetes, hypertension, and vascular disease, can also affect tissue oxygenation and increase the prevalence of fibrosis. Fibrosis is generally permanent, and the severity may increase with further follow-up. Clinical signs can include cutaneous induration, lymphedema, joint restriction, ulcerations, atrophy, telangiectasia, and photosensitivity.[5] Skin and soft tissue necrosis is generally managed with supportive care. A combination of pentoxifylline (PTX) and vitamin E has been examined for treatment of fibrosis. Initial studies in swine models demonstrated an approximate 50% decrease in the dimensions of fibrosis.[6] This was confirmed in a small study of breast

Table 1
Normal tissue tolerance to therapeutic irradiation: clinical endpoints and possible management strategies

Organ	TD 5/5 (Dose in Gy)	TD 50/5 (Dose in Gy)	Clinical Endpoint	Management Considerations
Kidneys	23–50	28–40	Nephritis	Expectant/dialysis
Bladder	65–80	80–85	Bladder contracture/volume loss/refractory hematuria	Consider hyperbaric oxygen (HBO)
Bladder			Acute cystitis/spasm	Analgesics (eg, phenazopyridine) and/or antispasmodics (eg, oxybutynin)
Femoral head	52	65	Necrosis	—
Skin	55–70	70	Necrosis, ulceration	Wound/burn management (silvadene, antibiotics, skin grafting if severe)
Skin			Acute desquamation	Moisturizing creams, hydrocortisone cream, hydrogel wound dressing, consider empiric antibiotics
Bone (mandible)			Osteoradionecrosis	Surgical debridement, antibiotics, consider HBO
Oral mucosa	60	75	Ulceration, fibrosis, mucositis	Wound care, oral hygiene and baking soda mouthwash, gelclair, narcotics, topical anesthetics, consider empiric antifungal
Brain	45–60	60–75	Necrosis, infarction	Corticosteroids, mannitol, neurosurgical evaluation
Spinal cord	47–50	70	Myelitis, necrosis	HBO questionable, high-dose steroids questionable
Brachial plexus	60–62	75–77	Plexopathy, nerve damage	HBO questionable, high-dose steroids questionable, physical therapy

Organ			Endpoint	Management
External/middle ear	30–55	40–65	Acute/chronic serous otitis	Earwax removal (Debrox), pseudoephedrine, myringotomy in severe cases
Parotid	32	46	Xerostomia	Pilocarpine, artificial saliva, antibacterial mouthwash, dental gum
Lung	18–45	25–65	Pneumonitis	Corticosteroids, antibiotics
Heart	40–60	50–70	Pericarditis	Corticosteroids, nonsteroidal anti-inflammatory
Esophagus	55–60	68–72	Stricture, perforation	Dilation
Esophagus			Acute esophagitis	Oral anesthetic solutions (eg, viscous lidocaine + benadryl or sucralfate suspension), soft diet, consider empiric antifungal
Prostate			Urinary irritative/obstructive symptoms	Alpha-1 blocker, anti-inflammatory, phenazopyridine (caution with antispasmodics)
Stomach	50–60	65–70	Ulceration, perforation	Surgical management
Small intestine	40–50	55–60	Obstruction, perforation, fistula	Surgical management
Colon	45–55	55–65	Obstruction, perforation, fistula	Surgical management
Rectum	60	80	Proctitis	Mesalamine, sulfasalazine, sucralfate enema, steroid suppositories

Adapted from Emami B, Lyman J, Brown A, et al. Tolerance of normal tissue to therapeutic irradiation. Int J Radiat Oncol Biol Phys 1991;21(1):109–22; with permission.

cancer patients given 800 mg/d of PTX and 1000 U/d of Vitamin E. A statistically significant regression in radiation-induced fibrosis was noted in patients taking both medications for 6 months. Nevertheless, the authors concluded that these results require confirmation in a larger study.[7] Longitudinal studies suggest that a long duration of therapy (12–24 months) is required for maximal regression of fibrosis.[8] Hyperbaric oxygen (HBO) treatment may also be effective for soft tissue necrosis. In one review of 23 patients with soft tissue or bony necrosis of the chest wall, HBO was an important adjunct to surgical debridement, with or without flap placement, and improvement was noted in the majority of patients.[9]

Pulmonary Toxicity

The pulmonary toxic effects of RT can have devastating and longstanding consequences, and this risk must be considered during treatment planning for lung cancer, breast cancer, and other thoracic malignancies. Pulmonary toxicity often presents with an acute inflammatory phase, which may be self-limited and improve with supportive measures, although severe cases may prove fatal. The later onset of RT-related pulmonary fibrosis (PF), which includes fibroblast proliferation and the destruction of normal lung architecture, has more lasting consequences.

Acute pulmonary toxicity that occurs in a previously radiated lung is referred to as radiation pneumonitis (RP). RP generally occurs within 1 to 3 months following completion of RT.[10,11] The underlying etiology and pathophysiology of RP are related to a cytokine-mediated signal cascade with proinflammatory and profibrotic factors.[10,12] Some preclinical studies suggest a role for transforming growth factor beta (TGF-β) and interleukin-6 (IL-6) as well as other cytokines in the development of RP.[10,12,13] Important factors in determining the risk of RP include volume of lung irradiated, the dose per RT fraction (to functioning lung), and the use of concurrent or sequential chemotherapy. Although several metrics have been evaluated to predict for RP, the V20, or volume of lung receiving at least 20 Gy, is the most frequently used parameter. Baseline poor pulmonary capacity and smoking may predict an increased risk of RP.[14] Individualized biologic factors are important, and serum TGF-β levels may help identify patients at risk of RP. A study from Duke University was successfully able to escalate the RT dose in patients who had lower TGF-β levels.[15]

The diagnosis of RP is generally made with an appropriate clinical history in a patient who has undergone previous RT to the chest (ie, lung cancer, breast cancer, or lymphoma). The differential diagnosis includes infectious pneumonia, pulmonary embolism, and tumor recurrence.[10,12] The diagnosis of RP may be particularly challenging in lung cancer patients who are at risk for pulmonary compromise due to severe underlying pulmonary dysfunction. Clinical symptoms are nonspecific and include cough (nonproductive or productive of clear sputum), low-grade fever, dyspnea, fatigue, and pleuritic chest pain.[11,12] Physical examination may reveal crackles or a pleural rub. Imaging very early on in the course of RP may not show abnormalities. Ground-glass opacities that conform to the RT port[11] classically define RP, although this is not a consistent finding.[11,16] In some patients, a lymphocytic alveolitis involving both adjacent lobes in the ipsilateral lung as well as the contralateral lung has been described after undergoing RT.[16] Symptoms are similar to RP, but radiographically, more diffuse changes are noted. A typical example of acute RP is shown in **Fig. 1**.

Single-photon emission computed tomography ventilation and perfusion scans can detect regional RT-induced lung injury (RILI) even at modest doses of RT.[12,17] Pulmonary-function tests (PFTs) may be diminished, although the diffusing capacity of carbon monoxide is preferentially affected.[12,14,18] A restrictive pattern is likely to emerge on PFTs in the late fibrotic phase. The cornerstone of management of acute

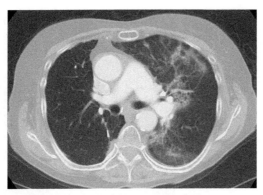

Fig. 1. Radiation pneumonitis: Computed tomographic (CT) scan.

RP is the use of high-dose corticosteroids. A dose of 30 to 60 mg/d of prednisone or 16 to 20 mg/d of dexamethasone should be started once the diagnosis of RILI is established.[19] Others have advocated a prednisone dose of 1 mg/kg/d.[20] Steroids should be gradually tapered over a period of weeks (reduce daily dose by ~10 mg/wk) to avoid flare-ups of RP.[19] Supplemental oxygen should be administered if indicated, and the differential diagnosis of infectious pneumonia must be considered. Symptoms of acute RP will generally improve over a matter of weeks to months with supportive management.

Several agents have shown promise in either reducing the risk of RP or treating RP. Clinical and preclinical studies have assessed captopril, cyclosporin, and PTX, amifostine, keratinocyte growth factor, and inhibitors of TGF-β. Amifostine has demonstrated variable effects in clinical studies but must be administered concurrently with thoracic RT to be effective.[21] Captopril, an angiotensin-converting enzyme inhibitor, is a thiol compound that can scavenge free radicals and stimulate IL-2. It has been found to reduce the incidence of RT-induced fibrosis in rats,[22] although extrapolation from this animal data suggests that much higher doses would be required for tissue protection than those administered for hypertension. A National Cancer Institute phase II randomized trial is currently underway to assess its efficacy.[20] Preclinical research involving a novel inhibitor of the TGF-β 1 receptor has demonstrated a decreased incidence in functional lung damage, inflammatory response, and serum TGF-β level.[22,23]

In the late setting, PF predominates.[9] PF generally occurs beyond 6 months.[10] The underlying pathophysiology is similar to fibrosis that occurs in other tissues, with pro-fibrotic cytokines, such as TGF-β IL-1 and IL-6, playing a role.[10,11] Chemotherapy with well-known agents, such as actinomycin D, adriamycin, bleomycin, busulfan, cyclophosphamide, and bis-chloronitrosourea, may exacerbate PF.[19] Many patients who previously received RT to the chest will have radiographic abnormalities, which may persist indefinitely, without exhibiting clinical symptoms. It is necessary to compare serial x-rays (if available) in patients who have a history of RT treatment to the chest to avoid misinterpreting chronic radiation changes as an acute process. An example of chronic radiation-induced fibrosis is shown in **Fig. 2**. Clinically significant RT-induced fibrosis may result in progressive chronic dyspnea;[11] however, there is no correlation between the extent of radiographic change and clinical symptoms.[10,11] Although current treatment is primarily supportive, ongoing research is evaluating the potential for several growth factor inhibitors to reverse PF.

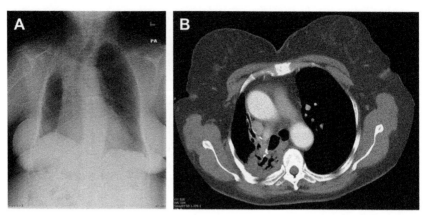

Fig. 2. Late radiation-associated PF and volume loss 7 y after treatment: (*A*) Chest x-ray. (*B*) Computed tomographic (CT) scan.

Endobronchial (intraluminal) brachytherapy (EBBT) is generally used in patients who have relapsed and/or have persistent airway tumors. Patients often have already received full-dose external beam RT. Even in patients with recurrent lesions, EBBT is effective in relieving symptoms such as dyspnea, hemoptysis, and postobstructive pneumonitis.[24] Massive, sometimes fatal, hemoptysis is a feared severe complication in patients undergoing EBBT. The largest series report fatal hemoptysis rates of 9% to 11%, and patients with tumors located in the main bronchi or upper lobes (possible close relationship to the pulmonary vasculature) were more likely to develop this complication.[24,25]

Stereotactic body radiation therapy (SBRT) involves the delivery of a few (< = 5) intense fractions of RT to a limited volume using advanced technologies. One of the most active areas of SBRT is in the treatment of patients with early stage nonsmall cell lung cancer who are unable to undergo surgical lobectomy. Although excellent rates of tumor control have been reported in several studies, there is an increased risk of severe pulmonary toxicity following treatment of centrally located (eg, peihilar) tumors due to resultant airway obstruction and atelectasis.[26] Radiographic changes are more severe than those seen with typical fractionated RT due to the ablative nature of SBRT. Another complication that is increasingly recognized in the treatment of peripheral lung lesions is rib pain and fracture. Treatment is typically supportive with analgesic medications.

Central Nervous System Toxicity

The risk of toxicity from CNS RT must be weighed against often dire consequences of tumor relapse in the brain. The underlying pathophysiology of acute neurocognitive change generally relates to radiation-induced disruption of the blood-brain barrier, which in and of itself may lead to increased toxicity when concurrent or adjuvant chemotherapy is used. The blood-brain barrier is disrupted secondary to endothelial cell damage, whereas glial cell damage can further contribute to neurotoxicity. Factors important in predicting long-term and short-term CNS toxic effects of RT include the RT volume, dose, fraction schedule, use of concurrent or sequential chemotherapy, and age of the patient (with extremes of age being more susceptible to toxicity).

Common acute side effects, which occur within a few weeks of beginning cranial RT, generally include mild fatigue, skin erythema, and alopecia. Radiation dermatitis,

when it does occur, is usually mild and can be ameliorated with the use of topical oint-
ments (eg, RadiaCare or Aquaphor). Nausea and headache are common in patients
undergoing cranial RT and may be secondary to mild cerebral edema. The administration of oral steroids (eg, Decadron in divided daily doses) and antinausea medication is
usually effective management.

Patients who have elevated intracranial pressure (ICP) and received large-volume
RT with a large fraction size (>3 Gy) are at risk for acute encephalopathy. Symptoms
can include nausea and vomiting, headache, somnolence, fever, and focal neurologic
deficits. It is important to realize that tumor-associated edema can cause many of the
same side effects, and if symptomatic cerebral edema is present, corticosteroids may
be indicated before beginning RT. In rare cases, cerebral herniation, or even death,
can occur.[19]

A serous otitis media with mucosal vasodilation and Eustachian tube edema may
occur after RT. In occasional cases, this may lead to tinnitus and high-frequency
hearing loss requiring myringotomy tubes, and, in extreme cases, cochlear implants
may be required.[27] Excessive cerumen buildup may occur within weeks to months
after completing RT and can be treated with gentle earwax removal kits such as
carbamide peroxide (Debrox) ear drops.

The somnolence syndrome includes symptoms of increased ICP, such as headache, nausea, vomiting, and irritability. The syndrome occurs most commonly in children who have previously undergone prophylactic whole-brain RT and is rare in
adults.[28–30] There are no radiographic or laboratory findings that are specific to the
diagnosis, and the syndrome is self-limited and usually resolves within 2 to 3 weeks.
Corticosteroids may improve symptoms in patients with this syndrome, although their
routine use is not recommended.[29]

Transient myelopathy may occur 2 to 4 months after spinal irradiation and may
present with Lhermitte's sign, which consists of an unpleasant electric shock-like
sensation that radiates down the spine and frequently into the limbs.[31] The symptoms
are precipitated by flexion of the neck[19] and are thought to be due to transient demye-
linization of the cord. Transient radiation myelopathy of the spinal cord is a clinical
diagnosis without specific radiographic findings. The syndrome is self-limiting, lasting
approximately 4 months on average, and does not require specific treatment and
generally does not predict permanent neurologic compromise.

Radiation necrosis of the brain can occur months to years after RT. The etiology is
vascular endothelial cell damage with resultant coagulative necrosis and demyelination secondary to chronic hypoxia.[32] Radiation necrosis generally develops in the
high-dose region of RT, with symptoms dependent on the location of the lesion. Focal
neurologic deficits and/or signs of increased ICP can occur. Conventional magnetic
resonance imaging (MRI) findings include a contrast-enhancing mass with
white-matter changes and/or edema. Magnetic resonance spectroscopy and fluorodeoxyglucose positron emission tomography imaging may help differentiate tumor
recurrence from necrosis,[33] although pathologic confirmation may be necessary.
The symptoms of radiation necrosis may be improved with corticosteroids and/or
mannitol, although surgical decompression may be required. Experience treating radiation necrosis with anticoagulation and HBO is limited.[34,35]

Nonspecific, diffuse white matter changes occur in the vast majority of patients
receiving conventional full-dose RT (in the case of gliomas, for example). Symptoms
of leukoencephalopathy can occur in both children and adults and were first described
in pediatric patients receiving prophylactic cranial RT and methotrexate for
leukemia.[36] Initial symptoms may include lethargy and seizures and, in some cases,
may progress to ataxia, overt confusion, dementia, and even death.[37] Differentiating

adverse effects of cranial RT from the effects of the underlying malignancy can be difficult. Data from studies involving the use of methylphenidate as well as the acetylcholinesterase inhibitor donepezil suggest a benefit to both drugs in improving long-term NCF in patients who have undergone cranial RT.[38,39] The herb ginkgo biloba is also the focus of an ongoing study.[40]

Radiation myelopathy is an uncommon late complication of spinal RT. The initial symptoms can include paresthesias and sensory changes, such as a decrease in proprioception or temperature sensation. These symptoms begin anywhere from 9 to 15 months after completion of RT.[41] Progressive symptoms may include altered bowel and bladder function, lower-extremity weakness, hyperreflexia, and, in some cases, a Brown-Séquard syndrome. Chronic radiation myelopathy, in contrast to the transient form, is generally irreversible. Similar to transient myelopathy, this is a diagnosis of exclusion, and a thorough differential diagnosis, including tumor recurrence, demyelinating diseases, and neurotoxicity secondary to iatrogenic causes, should be considered. A spinal MRI with gadolinium may be helpful in establishing the diagnosis. An MRI may show cord atrophy or swelling, decreased intensity on T1 images, and increased intensity on the T2 sequence, frequently with contrast enhancement.[42] There is no definite evidence of an effective therapy for chronic progressive radiation myelopathy. Interventions such as HBO, heparin, and warfarin have been tried, but only anecdotal evidence exists for these measures.[34,43] Ongoing research is assessing the role of stimulating growth factors, including platelet-derived growth factor, insulin-like growth factor, vascular endothelial growth factor, and basic fibroblast growth factor, in treating radiation myelitis.[44]

Hypothalamic and pituitary dysfunction commonly occur in both children and adults following RT.[45] Growth hormone production is the most sensitive to RT, more so than adrenalcorticotropic hormone or thyrotropin-releasing hormone. Children are especially susceptible to effects of cranial RT, with a variable time course of endocrine dysfunction after receiving treatment.

Head and Neck Toxicity

RT is frequently employed as a primary treatment for early stage head and neck cancer (HNC) and often combined with chemotherapy for more advanced-stage tumors. Chemotherapy potentiates both the beneficial and toxic effects of RT. Severe acute reactions often expected during RT include mucositis, dysphagia, odynophagia, xerostomia, dermatitis, and voice changes. Tumor- and patient-related factors are important in predicting acute toxicity, and social factors (eg, current and/or prior history of alcohol/tobacco abuse, poor dentition, malnutrition) as well as underlying medical comorbidities may exacerbate toxicity.

Oral mucositis results from the radiation-induced mitotic death of basal cells of the oral mucosal epithelium.[46] The superficial layers of the oral mucosa are lost through normal physiologic sloughing. The subsequent denuding of the epithelium results in mucositis. Characteristic symptoms of mucositis may include erythema, edema, tenderness, pain, dysphagia, and hoarseness. Mucositis typically manifests 2 to 3 weeks after beginning RT. Oral hygiene, dietary modification, and maintenance of nutritional status are integral to the management of mucositis. Avoidance of spicy or acidic foods, caffeine, tobacco, and alcohol will help symptomatic patients. Prophylactic placement of a gastric feeding tube should be considered. Topical anesthetics, often in combination with diphenhydramine or an antacid, are used during treatment for patients who develop painful mucositis and esophagitis. A "BMX" solution consisting of 1% to 2% viscous lidocaine, diphenhydramine, and Maalox provides short-term relief for oral intake. Care should be taken with the use of lidocaine-containing solutions, since anesthetized mucosa is more susceptible to trauma. Topical non-Rx gel protectants, such as benzocaine (Oratect) gel and GEL-CLAIR bioadherent oral gel (Helsinn Healthcare SA, Lugano, Switzerland), may provide a temporary protective barrier for inflamed mucosa before eating. Opioids (long acting and short acting) may be indicated for pain control in patients with severe mucositis, and transdermal fentanyl can be considered in patients unable to swallow oral medication. Mucositis will generally begin to resolve within a few weeks following the completion of RT.

Xerostomia related to salivary gland dysfunction is a common permanent effect of RT for HNC. Oral hygiene is critical, because decreased saliva production increases the risk of dental decay. Patients should frequently rinse and gargle with a solution of baking soda, salt, and water to help break up thickened oral secretions. Saliva substitutes have met with variable success and acceptance, and some patients will routinely carry a bottle of water with them. Amifostine, a sulfhydryl agent, is a free radical scavenger that has been shown to reduce the incidence of acute and chronic xerostomia in patients receiving conventional RT as well as chemoradiation for HNC.[47,48] Pilocarpine, a cholinergic agent, has also been examined as an agent to reduce xerostomia. It is generally given 5 mg 3 times a day during RT and thereafter. In one study, there was an increased rate of salivary function in the pilocarpine-treated group compared with that in the placebo, but the benefit on quality of life was unclear.[49]

Patients undergoing RT for HNC are prone to develop oral candidiasis, which can exacerbate mucositis.[46] Treatment of oral candidiasis can be accomplished through either the use of topical antifungal medication (eg, Nystatin "swish and swallow") or systemic antifungal medication (eg, fluconazole), which may be better tolerated in patients experiencing severe mucositis.

The unilateral blood supply to each half of the mandible can predispose patients to osteoradionecrosis (ORN). ORN typically presents within 3 years after completion of RT for HNC. ORN can present with a variety of symptoms, including pain, loss of sensation, fistula, halitosis, trismus, pathologic fracture, or infection. The diagnosis of ORN generally relies on clinical examination of chronically exposed bone. Radiographic findings include decreased bone density and pathologic fractures. The incidence of ORN based on retrospective studies ranges from 0.4% to 56%, with one of the largest series reporting an incidence of 8.2%.[50] The most common location for ORN is the body of mandible. Tooth extractions following RT are a common precipitant to ORN,[50] and HBO protocols may be considered before extraction in patients at risk.[46] Mild ORN is generally managed conservatively with debridement, therapeutic ultrasound, and antibiotics.[51] When there is extensive bone and soft tissue necrosis, radical resection with immediate microvascular reconstruction is indicated.[52] HBO is generally recommended for the management of ORN, in that it increases oxygenation of irradiated tissue, promotes angiogenesis, enhances osteoblast repopulation, and fibroblast function.[46] If surgery is used to manage ORN, traditionally, 10 dives of post-surgical HBO were recommended.[53] More recent protocols generally call for 30 preoperative HBO sessions at 2.4 atm for 90 minutes each, followed by 10 treatments after surgery.[54] Before HBO therapy was available, reconstruction of previously irradiated mandibular tissue in patients with oropharyngeal and other head and neck tumors was often unsuccessful, with complications, including osteonecrosis, soft tissue radionecrosis, mucositis, dermatitis, and laryngeal radionecrosis, developing in 50% to 60% of patients. With HBO, success rates of up to 93% have been reported among selected patients.[55] In severe cases of ORN, partial mandibulectomy may be required.

Dysphagia and pharyngeal dysfunction are to be expected in patients receiving chemotherapy and RT in HNC. Radiation of the oropharynx can lead to edema, fibrosis, and, in rare cases, pharyngeal stenosis. One study examined serial swallowing studies (fluoroscopy and esophagograms) performed pretherapy, 1 to 3 months post-RT and 6 to 12 months post-RT. Post-treatment changes included reduced inversion of the cricopharyngeal muscle and laryngeal closure, promoting aspiration.[54] Oropharyngeal strictures can be treated with balloon dilation, but they frequently recur. Severe pharyngeal/laryngeal edema that develops during a course of RT can interfere with respiration in extreme cases and may require tracheostomy.[55] Hoarseness may result from RT to the laryngeal structures and generally improves with time, although continued smoking after treatment is associated with persistent hoarseness.[56]

Toxic Effects of Abdominal and Pelvic Radiotherapy

The liver may be irradiated during treatment of lower-lobe lung cancers, esophageal tumors, stomach cancer, pancreatic malignancies, and lymphomas, in addition to primary liver tumors. RT-associated liver toxicity may present similarly to hepatitis with vague right upper quadrant abdominal pain progressing to hepatomegaly and ascites. Anicteric ascites generally occurs a few months after RT, although the onset can occur more rapidly after chemoradiation.[19] Alkaline phosphatase is usually increased in radiation hepatopathy. Chronic hepatitis and cirrhosis associated with RT are mediated by TGF-β, similar to radiation-associated PF.[57] The characteristic lesion seen in late radiation hepatopathy is central venous occlusive disease, which is characterized by retrograde congestion on liver biopsy. Veno-occlusive lesions can appear as early as 2.5 months after a patient undergoes RT. The differential diagnosis includes other causes of liver disease, such as infectious hepatitis, metastatic disease, and drug-induced hepatitis. Treatment is primarily supportive, although transplant may be considered in select cases of severe radiation hepatopathy.

The small and large intestine are vulnerable portions of the GI tract and can undergo radiation-associated enteritis. Acute GI symptoms that occur within a few weeks of starting RT include increased stool frequency and loss of form, with eventual diarrhea. This is generally self-limiting and occurs as the result of acute mucosal changes after the initiation of RT. These effects may be exacerbated by the coadministration of chemotherapy agents. The mucosa is rapidly renewed, limiting the duration of these acute effects. Gentle use of antidiarrheals can be considered in addition to dietary modification. Late effects of the GI tract, including stricture and ulceration, can occur secondary to radiation endarteritis and chronic ischemia. Ulceration and infarction necrosis can occur with rapid obliteration of the vessels, whereas fibrosis, strictures, and fistulas may form due to more gradual narrowing of the finer vasculature. Surgical handling of irradiated bowel must be performed cautiously due to the tenuous blood supply to limit further vascular dysfunction and injury. The differential diagnosis must include small-bowel obstruction in patients with prior abdominal surgery, whether or not RT has been given.

Acute radiation-associated proctitis is generally self-limiting, with symptoms such as diarrhea, rectal urgency, and, rarely, bleeding, resolving within a few months.[58] Chronic or late radiation proctitis generally occurs 1 to 2 years after undergoing RT and is due to epithelial atrophy and fibrosis associated with the obliterative "endarteritis" seen in other late radiation toxicity syndromes. Symptoms associated with chronic radiation proctitis include diarrhea, obstructed defecation (secondary to stricture development), bleeding, tenesmus, and, occasionally, fecal incontinence. Diagnosis of chronic radiation proctitis is based on the clinical history, confirmed with findings found on colonoscopy or sigmoid-oscopy. Changes to the mucosa can include pallor with friability and telangiecta-sias.[59] Mucosal biopsies can assess for other causes of proctitis such as inflammatory bowel disorders, although they must be performed with the utmost care, as radiated tissue is more prone to fistula formation and chronic nonhealing ulcerations.[60] Treatment should be directed at symptom management. Dietary assessment is critical, and the routine use of stool softeners and/or fiber additives may be valuable in patients suffering from constipation. In patients with mild symptoms, such as a small amount of intermittent rectal bleeding, anti-inflamma-tory suppositories (eg, hydrocortisone, mesalamine) may be beneficial. Symptoms can resolve spontaneously in up to a third of patients.[61] Refractory rectal bleeding should be assessed by colonoscopy to assess for other causes. Sulfasalazine has also been used either in oral or enema preparations with some success. Steroids, such as prednisolone, that have been added to these preparations have demon-strated further efficacy.[62] Topical sucralfate (given twice a day as an enema) also shows some efficacy in small clinical studies and may be more efficacious than combination sulfasalazine/prednisolone.[62]

Acute genitourinary effects of RT to the bladder and urethra include urinary frequency, urgency, and irritation. These effects are exacerbated when concomitant chemotherapy is used. Incontinence is rarely observed in the acute period in patients who were continent before the initiation of therapy. General management includes urinary anesthetic agents and antispasmotics. Urinary tract infections may coexist and should be considered in cases of persistent or refractory symptoms. Dietary modification, particularly with the elimination of caffeine and alcohol, may help to mini-mize symptoms. In men who have been treated for prostate cancer with brachyther-apy, there is a 5% to 15% risk of urinary retention due to prostate edema.[63] If possible, men should be taught how to perform intermittent self-catheterization rather than having an indwelling catheter. Urinary retention will generally resolve within a matter of weeks. Care should be taken to assess amount of residual urine in the bladder, as the administration of antispasmodics (eg, oxybutynin [Ditropan]) may precipitate urinary retention. Medication with alpha blockers (eg, tamsulosin [Flomax]) should be considered in men who have obstructive symptoms. Transurethral resection of the prostate after RT is associated with an increased risk of incontinence and should only be considered in men who are refractory to conservative measures. Acute urinary irritative symptoms generally resolve (or greatly improve) within 3 to 6 weeks following the completion of external beam RT but may persist for several months in men treated with permanent seed implant.

Late genitourinary complications of RT include persistent irritative voiding symp-toms. Urinary incontinence may be precipitated or exacerbated, particularly in men who are postprostatectomy. Severe late radiation cystitis and hematuria may occur in 3% to 5% of patients. This requires evaluation by cystoscopy, as hematuria may also signify the presence of bladder cancer recurrence. Moreover, men who have received RT for prostate cancer are at increased risk for developing secondary bladder cancer. Hematuria that is refractory to conservative measures can be effec-tively treated with HBO. In one study of 57 patients with radiation-induced hemor-rhagic cystitis (mean time, 48 months from completion of RT), 86% had either complete resolution or marked improvement after HBO.[64] Urethral stricture and bladder neck contracture occur in less than 5% of patients, but the risk is increased in patients treated with combined surgery and RT. Treatment with outpatient urethral dilation is generally successful in alleviating symptoms, although repeat dilations may be necessary.

Cardiac Toxicity

A spectrum of cardiac injury can occur when the heart is irradiated. Late effects are most common due to radiation-induced vascular damage and endarteritis. Acute effects, such as pericarditis, may be observed after treatment of a substantial volume of the entire heart, such as in selected cases of Hodgkin's lymphoma (HL), but this is relatively uncommon. Long-term effects include coronary artery disease (CAD), cardiomyopathy, valvular damage, and dysrhythmias. These effects generally manifest years to decades after the original course of RT. CAD may appear 10 to 15 years after RT but is also affected by the patient's underlying cardiac risk factors, including obesity, diabetes, smoking, hypertension, and family history. High-risk populations include those with breast cancer and HL, many of whom were treated at a young enough age to manifest chronic radiation toxicity several years later.

The hallmarks of late radiation-associated cardiotoxicity include diffuse fibrosis of the myocardial interstitium with narrowing of the arterial and capillary lumens. Eventually, the number of capillaries is reduced relative to the number of myocytes, leading to ischemia, cell death, and replacement with collagen and fibrin.[65] CAD results from injury to the intima of the cardiac endothelium in a cascade of events that is typical of atherosclerosis, including deposition of platelets and myofibroblasts along with replacement of the damaged intima.[65] Fibrosis can occur in the cusp and/or leaflets of the valves as well as the wall of the ventricles, affecting cardiac compliance and contractility.[66] Dysrhythmias can arise when fibrosis occurs within the conduction system.[67] HL patients who have been treated with RT have an increased risk of valvular heart disease.[68] Mortality from myocardial infarction is also increased in patients with HL, mainly in those who were treated with anthracycline-based chemotherapy or supradiaphragmatic RT.[69–71]

SUMMARY

Radiation oncologists and emergency department physicians must be familiar with the underlying pathophysiology of RT-induced normal tissue toxicity, particularly in the context of multimodality therapy. Although most acute toxicities will be managed by the oncology team, many patients presenting to the emergency department will have a history of cancer treatment including RT. A better appreciation and understanding of the acute and late toxicities associated with RT will help improve the medical decision making in these patients. Advances in radiation oncology technology coupled with an improved understanding of the underlying biology of toxic reactions should result in fewer severe complications in the future.

REFERENCES

1. Khan FM. Interactions of ionizing radiation. In: The Physics of radiation therapy. Philadelphia: Lippincott Williams & Wilkins; 2003. p. 59–61.
2. Hall EJ, Giaccia EJ. Physics and chemistry of radiation absorption. In: Radiobiology for the radiologist. Philadelphia: Lippincott Williams & Wilkins; 2006. p. 5–14.
3. Hall EJ, Giaccia EJ. Clinical response of normal tissues. In: Radiobiology for the radiologist. Philadelphia: Lippincott Williams & Wilkins; 2006. p. 327–44.
4. Goodman M, Hilderly LJ, Purl S. Integumentary and mucous membrane alterations. In: Groenwald SL, Goodman M, Yarbro CH, editors. Cancer nursing principles and practice. 4th edition. Boston (MA): Jones and Bartlett; 1997. p. 768–822.

5. Wood G, Casey L, Trotti A. Skin changes. In: Small W, Woloschak GE, editors. Radiation toxicity: a practical guide. New York: Springer Science; 2006. p. 170–81.

6. Lefaix JL, Delanian S, Vozenin MC, et al. Striking regression of subcutaneous fibrosis induced by high doses of gamma rays using a combination of pentoxifylline and alpha-tocopherol: an experimental study. Int J Radiat Oncol Biol Phys 1999;43(4):839–47.

7. Delanian S, Porcher R, Balla-Mekias S, et al. Randomized, placebo-controlled trial of combined pentoxifylline and tocopherol for regression of superficial radiation-induced fibrosis. J Clin Oncol 2003;21(13):2545–50.

8. Delanian S, Porcher R, Rudant J, et al. Kinetics of response to long-term treatment combining pentoxifylline and tocopherol in patients with superficial radiation-induced fibrosis. J Clin Oncol 2005;23(34):8570–9.

9. Feldmeier JJ, Heimbach RD, Davolt DA, et al. Hyperbaric oxygen as an adjunctive treatment for delayed radiation injury of the chest wall: a retrospective review of twenty-three cases. Undersea Hyperb Med 1995;22(4): 383–93.

10. Chen Y, Williams J, Ding I, et al. Radiation pneumonitis and early circulatory cytokine markers. Semin Radiat Oncol 2002;12(1 Suppl 1):26–33.

11. Monson JM, Stark P, Reilly JJ. Clinical radiation pneumonitis and radiographic changes after thoracic radiation therapy for lung carcinoma. Cancer 1998; 82(5):842–50.

12. Marks LB, Yu X, Vujaskovic Z, et al. Radiation-induced lung injury. Semin Radiat Oncol 2003;13(3):333–45.

13. Anscher MS, Kong FM, Andrews K, et al. Plasma transforming growth factor beta1 as a predictor of radiation pneumonitis. Int J Radiat Oncol Biol Phys 1998;41(5):1029–35.

14. Smith LM, Mendenhall NP, Cicale MJ, et al. Results of a prospective study evaluating the effects of mantle irradiation on pulmonary function. Int J Radiat Oncol Biol Phys 1989;16(1):79–84.

15. Anscher MS, Marks LB, Shafman TD, et al. Risk of long-term complications after TFG-beta1-guided very-high-dose thoracic radiotherapy. Int J Radiat Oncol Biol Phys 2003;56(4):988–95.

16. Arbetter KR, Prakash UB, Tazelaar HD, et al. Radiation-induced pneumonitis in the "nonirradiated" lung. Mayo Clin Proc 1999;74(1):27–36.

17. Rodrigues G, Lock M, D'Souza D, et al. Prediction of radiation pneumonitis by dose - volume histogram parameters in lung cancer–a systematic review. Radiother Oncol 2004;71(2):127–38.

18. Brady LW, Germon PA, Cander L. The effects of radiation therapy on pulmonary function in carcinoma in the Lung. Radiology 1965;85:130–4.

19. Constine LS, Milano MT, Friedman D, et al. Late effects of cancer treatment on normal tissues. In: Halperin EC, Perez CA, Brady LW, editors. Perez and Brady's principles and practice of radiation oncology. 5th edition. Philadelphia: Lippincott Williams & Wilkins; 2007. p. 320–55.

20. Bradley J, Movsas B. Radiation pneumonitis and esophagitis in thoracic irradiation. In: Small W, Woloschak GE, editors. Radiation toxicity: a practical guide. New York: Springer Science; 2006. p. 42–53.

21. Komaki R, Lee JS, Milas L, et al. Effects of amifostine on acute toxicity from concurrent chemotherapy and radiotherapy for inoperable non-small-cell lung cancer: report of a randomized comparative trial. Int J Radiat Oncol Biol Phys 2004;58(5):1369–77.

22. Ward WF, Molteni A, Tsao CH. Radiation-induced endothelial dysfunction and fibrosis in rat lung: modification by the angiotensin converting enzyme inhibitor CL242817. Radiat Res 1989;117(2):342–50.

23. Anscher MS, Thrasher B, Zgonjanin L, et al. Small molecular inhibitor of transforming growth factor-beta protects against development of radiation-induced lung injury. Int J Radiat Oncol Biol Phys 2008;71(3):829–37.

24. Kelly JF, Delclos ME, Morice RC, et al. High-dose-rate endobronchial brachytherapy effectively palliates symptoms due to airway tumors: the 10-year M.D. Anderson cancer center experience. Int J Radiat Oncol Biol Phys 2000;48(3):697–702.

25. Ozkok S, Karakoyun-Celik O, Goksel T, et al. High dose rate endobronchial brachytherapy in the management of lung cancer: Response and toxicity evaluation in 158 patients. Lung Cancer 2008;62(3):326–33.

26. Timmerman R, McGarry R, Yiannoutsos C, et al. Excessive toxicity when treating central tumors in a phase II study of stereotactic body radiation therapy for medically inoperable early-stage lung cancer. J Clin Oncol 2006;24(30): 4833–9.

27. Jereczek-Fossa BA, Zarowski A, Milani F, et al. Radiotherapy-induced ear toxicity. Cancer Treat Rev 2003;29(5):417–30.

28. Freeman JE, Johnston PG, Voke JM. Somnolence after prophylactic cranial irradiation in children with acute lymphoblastic leukaemia. Br Med J 1973;4:523.

29. Uzal D, Ozyar E, Hayran M, et al. Reduced incidence of the somnolence syndrome after prophylactic cranial irradiation in children with acute lymphoblastic leukemia. Radiother Oncol 1998;48:29.

30. Schultheiss T, Kun L, Ang K, et al. Radiation response of the central nervous system. Int J Radiat Oncol Biol Phys 1995;31:1093.

31. Jones AM. Transient radiation myelopathy. Br J Radiol 1964;37(727):744.

32. Burger PC, Mahley MS Jr, Dudka L, et al. The morphologic effects of radiation administered therapeutically for intracranial gliomas: a postmortem study of 25 cases. Cancer 1979;44(4):1256–72.

33. Henry RG, Vigneron DB, Fischbein NJ, et al. Comparison of relative cerebral blood volume and proton spectroscopy in patients with treated gliomas. AJNR Am J Neuroradiol 2000;21(2):357–66.

34. Glantz MJ, Burger PC, Friedman AH, et al. Treatment of radiation-induced nervous system injury with heparin and warfarin. Neurology 1994;44(11):2020–7.

35. Chuba PJ, Aronin P, Bhambhani K, et al. Hyperbaric oxygen therapy for radiation-induced brain injury in children. Cancer 1997;80(10):2005–12.

36. Price RA, Jamieson PA. The central nervous system in childhood leukemia. II. Subacute leukoencephalopathy. Cancer 1975;35(2):306–18.

37. Frytak S, Shaw JN, O'Neill BP, et al. Leukoencephalopathy in small cell lung cancer patients receiving prophylactic cranial irradiation. Am J Clin Oncol 1989;12(1):27.

38. Mulhern RK, Khan RB, Kaplan S, et al. Short-term efficacy of methylphenidate: a randomized, double-blind, placebo-controlled trial among survivors of childhood cancer. J Clin Oncol 2004;22(23):4795–803.

39. Shaw EG, Rosdhal R, D'Agostino RB, et al. Phase II study of donepezil in irradiated brain tumor patients: effect on cognitive function, mood, and quality of life. J Clin Oncol 2006;24(9):1415–20.

40. Le Bars PL, Katz MM, Berman N. A placebo-controlled, double-blind, randomized trial of an extract of ginkgo biloba for dementia. JAMA 1997;278:1327–32.

41. Schultheiss TE, Higgins EM, El-Mahdi AM. The latent period in clinical radiation myelopathy. Int J Radiat Oncol Biol Phys 1984;10(7):1109–15.

42. Wang PY, Shen WC, Jan JS. Serial MRI changes in radiation myelopathy. Neuro-radiology 1995;37(5):374–7.
43. Luk KH, Baker DG, Fellows CF. Hyperbaric oxygen after radiation and its effect on the production of radiation myelitis. Int J Radiat Oncol Biol Phys 1978;4(5–6): 457–9.
44. Andratschke NH, Nieder C, Price RE, et al. Potential role of growth factors in di-minishing radiation therapy neural tissue injury. Semin Oncol 2005;32(2 Suppl 3): S67–70.
45. Constine LS, Woolf PD, Cann D, et al. Hypothalamic-pituitary dysfunction after radiation for brain tumors. N Engl J Med 1993;328(2):87–94.
46. Blanco AI, Chao C. Management of radiation-induced head and neck injury. In: Small W, Woloschak GE, editors. Radiation toxicity: a practical guide. New York: Springer Science; 2006. p. 23–39.
47. Büntzel J, Küttner K, Fröhlich D, et al. Selective cytoprotection with amifostine in concurrent radiochemotherapy for head and neck cancer. Ann Oncol 1998;9(5): 505–9.
48. Wasserman TH, Brizel DM, Henke M, et al. Influence of intravenous amifostine on xerostomia, tumor control, and survival after radiotherapy for head-and-neck cancer: 2-year follow-up of a prospective, randomized, phase III trial. Int J Radiat Oncol Biol Phys 2005;63(4):985–90.
49. Fisher J, Scott C, Scarantino CW. Phase III quality-of-life study results: impact on patients' quality of life to reducing xerostomia after radiotherapy for head-and-neck cancer–RTOG 97-09. Int J Radiat Oncol Biol Phys 2003;56(3):832–6.
50. Reuther T, T Schuster T, Mende U. Osteoradionecrosis of the jaws as a side effect of radiotherapy of head and neck tumour patients—a report of a thirty year retro-spective review. Int J Oral Maxillofac Surg 2003;32:289–95.
51. Wong JK, Wood RE, McLean M. Conservative management of osteoradionecro-sis. Oral Surg Oral Med Oral Pathol Oral Radiol Endod 1997;84(1):16–21.
52. Shaha AR, Cordeiro PG, Hidalgo DA, et al. Resection and immediate microvas-cular reconstruction in the management of osteoradionecrosis of the mandible. Head Neck 1997;19(5):406–11.
53. Marx RE, Ames JR. The use of hyperbaric oxygen therapy in bony reconstruction of the irradiated and tissue-deficient patient. J Oral Maxillofac Surg 1982;40(7): 412–20.
54. Tibbles PM, Edelsberg JS. Hyperbaric Oxygen Therapy. N Engl J Med 1996; 334(25):1642–8.
55. Hart GB, Mainous EG. The treatment of radiation necrosis with hyperbaric oxygen (OHP). Cancer 1976;37:2580–5.
56. Eisbruch A, Lyden T, Bradford CR, et al. Objective assessment of swallowing dysfunction and aspiration after radiation concurrent with chemotherapy for head-and-neck cancer. Int J Radiat Oncol Biol Phys 2002;53:23–8.
57. Lee HJ, Zelefsky MJ, Kraus DH, et al. Long-term regional control after radiation therapy and neck dissection for base of tongue carcinoma. Int J Radiat Oncol Biol Phys 1997;38(5):995–1000.
58. Verdonck-de Leeuw IM, Keus RB, Hilgers FJ, et al. Consequences of voice impairment in daily life for patients following radiotherapy for early glottic cancer: voice quality, vocal function, and vocal performance. Int J Radiat Oncol Biol Phys 1999;44(5):1071–8.
59. Anscher MS, Peters WP, Reisenbichler H, et al. Transforming growth factor beta as a predictor of liver and lung fibrosis after autologous bone marrow transplan-tation for advanced breast cancer. N Engl J Med 1993;328(22):1592–8.

60. Babb RR. Radiation proctitis: a review. Am J Gastroenterol 1996;91(7):1309–11.
61. O'Brien PC, Hamilton CS, Denham JW, et al. Spontaneous improvement in late rectal mucosal changes after radiotherapy for prostate cancer. Int J Radiat Oncol Biol Phys 2004;58(1):75–80.
62. Chrouser KL, Leibovich BC, Sweat SD, et al. Urinary fistulas following external radiation or permanent brachytherapy for the treatment of prostate cancer. J Urol 2005;173(6):1953–7.
63. Gilinsky NH, Burns DG, Barbezat GO, et al. The natural history of radiation-induced proctosigmoiditis: an analysis of 88 patients. QJM 1983;52(205):40–53 Winter.
64. Kochhar R, Patel F, Dhar A, et al. Radiation-induced proctosigmoiditis. Prospective, randomized, double-blind controlled trial of oral sulfasalazine plus rectal steroids versus rectal sucralfate. Dig Dis Sci 1991;36(1):103–7.
65. Bucci J, Morris WJ, Keyes M, et al. Predictive factors of urinary retention following prostate brachytherapy. Int J Radiat Oncol Biol Phys 2002;53(1):91–8.
66. Corman JM, McClure D, Pritchett R, et al. Treatment of radiation induced hemorrhagic cystitis with hyperbaric oxygen. J Urol 2003;169(6):2200–2.
67. Cuzick J, Stewart H, Rutqvist L, et al. Cause-specific mortality in long-term survivors of breast cancer who participated in trials of radiotherapy. J Clin Oncol 1994; 12(3):447–53.
68. Hardenbergh PH, Munley MT, Bentel GC, et al. Cardiac perfusion changes in patients treated for breast cancer with radiation therapy and doxorubicin: preliminary results. Int J Radiat Oncol Biol Phys 2001;49(4):1023–8.
69. Orzan F, Brusca A, Gaita F, et al. Associated cardiac lesions in patients with radiation-induced complete heart block. Int J Cardiol 1993;39(2):151–6.
70. Hull MC, Morris CG, Pepine CJ, et al. Valvular dysfunction and carotid, subclavian, and coronary artery disease in survivors of Hodgkin lymphoma treated with radiation therapy. JAMA 2003;290(21):2831–7.
71. Swerdlow AJ, Higgins CD, Smith P, et al. Myocardial infarction mortality risk after treatment for Hodgkin disease: a collaborative British cohort study. J Natl Cancer Inst 2007;99(3):206–14.

Management of Cancer-Related Pain

Paul L. DeSandre, DO[a], Tammie E. Quest, MD[b],*

KEYWORDS

- Pain • Malignant • Cancer • Opioids
- Emergency department

Patients and families struggling with cancer fear pain more than any other physical symptom. With the treatment of malignant pain remaining a challenge in the practice of oncology, the emergency department (ED) is often a place of refuge.[1] There are significant barriers to optimal pain management in the emergency setting, including lack of knowledge, inexperienced clinicians, myths about addiction, and fears of complications after discharge. These factors contribute to unnecessary suffering not only for the patient but also for family and caregivers. Malignant pain is highly responsive to medication. Adequate malignant pain control is possible in more than 90% of patients if established therapeutic approaches are applied systematically in any practice setting, including the ED.[2–7] It has been suggested that management of an acute pain crisis in a patient with advanced cancer "is as much a crisis as a code," and emergency clinicians should, and can, become comfortable caring for patients with cancer in acute pain.[8]

Patients with cancer often present to the ED because their pain is unmanageable. Although there are multiple physiologic possibilities for inadequate pain control, the emergency clinician should also be aware of the many psychosocial factors contributing to oligoanalgesia in the cancer patient. Depression, unresolved spiritual or social concerns, and misconceptions of prescribed medications may interfere with adequate treatment. With a properly focused evaluation, the treatment of unresolved pain in the cancer patient can be performed rapidly and effectively in the ED.

ASSESSMENT OF MALIGNANT PAIN

General principles of good pain assessment are particularly important in the patient presenting to the ED with malignancy. A rapid assessment of severity, character, likely

A version of this article was previously published in the *Emergency Medicine Clinics of North America*, 27:2.

[a] Department of Emergency Medicine, Beth Israel Medical Center, First Avenue, 16th Street, New York, NY 10003, USA

[b] Department of Emergency Medicine, Emory University School of Medicine, 69 Jesse Hill Jr Drive, Atlanta, GA 30303, USA

* Corresponding author.

E-mail address: tquest@emory.edu

Hematol Oncol Clin N Am 24 (2010) 643–658

doi:10.1016/j.hoc.2010.03.002

0889-8588/10/$ – see front matter © 2010 Elsevier Inc. All rights reserved.

etiology, timing and location, exacerbating and relieving factors, and associated symptoms provides essential information for proper management. In addition, the details of the history may reveal particular cancer pain syndromes, some of which require urgent diagnosis and intervention to prevent permanent functional impairment. With an adequate assessment, effective therapy can be quickly implemented in the ED.

The assessment of pain severity in cancer is the same as that of nonmalignant pain. There are several validated measures of a patient's pain experience. Although any scale is useful for a given patient as long as it is applied consistently, the preferred scale for most patients is the numerical rating scale (NRS).[9] Most commonly, this is an 11-point scale from 0 = "no pain" to 10 = "worst possible pain." For small children or patients with limited literacy, a picture scale is more successful, with the Faces Pain Scale being a well-accepted choice.[10] In the cognitively impaired patient, the 5-time observational Pain Assessment in Advanced Dementia Scale may be used.[11,12] All of these scales have been validated and have utility in the ED for the assessment of pain. It should be emphasized that pain scales are intended to provide objectivity to the experience of the patient's pain. Skepticism has no place in the assessment of suffering and may directly impair proper diagnosis and treatment. Pain can be complex, and these scales provide an objective method of evaluation to gauge treatment success. This is particularly true in acute pain.

The character and etiology of pain are described physiologically as either nociceptive or neuropathic. Cancer pain can be either or both. Nociceptive pain is a response to damaged tissue and can further be classified as either somatic (musculoskeletal/cutaneous) or visceral. Somatic pain is often described as sharp or aching and localized to the area of tissue damage. Pain secondary to bone metastasis is a classic example of somatic pain. Visceral pain is more poorly localized and can be intermittent, sometimes described as dull or cramping. Abdominal pain associated with ovarian or pancreatic cancers is characteristic. Neuropathic pain is primarily caused by nerve injury. The injury may be mechanical (eg, amputation), metabolic (eg, diabetes), inflammatory (eg, radiation), or toxic (eg, chemotherapy). Neuropathic pain is typically persistent and sometimes paroxysmal and shock-like. Normal stimulus may elicit abnormal pain responses (allodynia). A light touch, for example, may elicit searing pain. There can also be autonomic instability in the affected area, including edema or localized sweating such as that which occurs with complex reflex sympathetic dystrophy. An important treatment distinction between these types of pain is that patients with nociceptive pain are generally more responsive to opioids than are patients with neuropathic pain. Neuropathic pain often requires adjunctive nonopioid therapies for successful treatment.

Pain may rapidly change either in quality or location or may be chronic and slowly progressive. Although the alleviation of the pain crisis should always be the first priority, a search for the cause of the underlying pain ensures the most definitive treatment. Specific types of acute pain may require particular therapies for effective treatment, such as radiation therapy for bone metastasis. Likewise, a new location of pain may be the first sign of a dangerous progression of disease requiring diagnostic evaluation, such as new back pain preceding functional deficit in malignant epidural spinal cord compression. In addition to tumor progression, the aggressive treatments for malignancy may also be a cause for the patient's pain presentation. Surgical tumor resection may have predictable and self-limited associated pain, whereas chemotherapy-induced neuropathy may be less predictable and more persistent. The approach to treatment of these distinct types of pain will be quite different.

The assessment and management of chronic cancer pain (generally regarded as >3 months) can be challenging. Although similar to acute cancer pain in that either disease progression or treatment is typically responsible for the pain, these patients often carry a heavier global burden of suffering. The approach to treatment is more complex and must consider existing medications as well as other factors that may influence the approach to treatment.

Prior to diagnostic and therapeutic efforts in the ED, treatment must be guided by a clear understanding of the patient's goals of care. Some patients may not wish detailed investigations but may simply require pain treatment. Both acute and chronic cancer pain may be caused by disease progression (62%–78%), treatment (19%–25%), or unrelated (3%–10%) causes.[13] Patients who develop new pain are, therefore, reasonably anxious about disease progression. Communication should be sensitive to these concerns. The highly functional patient might have a goal of aggressively preserving function and longevity through early and aggressive diagnosis and management, whereas comfort alone may be the goal in an imminently dying patient.

The inescapable physical symptoms and the relentless awareness of the progression of the cancer contribute to physical, spiritual, social, and psychological strife. These factors all have the capacity to exacerbate the underlying pain. In addition, patients with pre-existing nonmalignant pain may come to the diagnosis of cancer already experiencing a sense of overwhelming suffering.[14] Cancer patients with pain are twice as likely to develop a psychiatric disorder, and as the disease progresses, the risk increases. The causes are multifactorial, and like pain, may be related to disease progression or treatment. Many of these disorders are amenable to treatment, which should be implemented as early as possible through proper referral and follow-up.[15] An interdisciplinary palliative care team, potentially hospice, should be involved as early as possible. Early palliative care intervention improves patient outcomes[16] and should be initiated by the emergency clinician when the need is identified. Depending on the institution and the urgency of the situation, palliative care consultation may occur in the ED, during hospitalization, or in the outpatient setting.

TREATMENT STRATEGIES
The WHO Stepladder

With a clear assessment of the details of the patient's pain, effective treatment can be rapidly implemented in the ED. In 1986 the WHO developed a 3-step ladder to guide the management of cancer pain. It was originally developed to address nociceptive pain (both somatic and visceral) but has proved useful to some degree for neuropathic pain as well. This simple and well-tested approach provides the clinician with a rational guide for the use of selected analgesics. Today, there is general consensus favoring the use of this model for all pain associated with serious illness. Management is based on the initial assessment of pain and should start at the step that corresponds to the patient's reported severity based on an NRS (0–10). Mild pain is defined as NRS 1 to 3 (step 1), moderate pain as NRS 4 to 6 (step 2), and severe pain as NRS 7 to 10 (step 3).

Step 1 analgesics
All of the nonopioid analgesics that characterize step 1 of the WHO ladder have a ceiling effect to their analgesia (a maximum dose that, if exceeded, yields no further analgesia). Acetaminophen is an effective step 1 analgesic and may be a useful coanalgesic in many situations, including headache. Its site and mechanism of action are not entirely known. It does not have significant anti-inflammatory effects and is presumed to have a central cyclo-oxygenase (COX) related mechanism. Chronic doses more than 4.0 g/24 h or acute doses more than 6.0 g/24 h are not

recommended because they may cause hepatotoxicity. Hepatic disease or heavy alcohol use increases the risk further, and the maximum daily dosage may be reduced to 3.0 g/24 h.

Nonsteroidal anti-inflammatory drugs (NSAIDs, including aspirin) are also effective step 1 analgesics and may be useful coanalgesics. They work, at least in part, by inhibiting COX, the enzyme that converts arachidonic acid to prostaglandins. There are several classes of NSAIDs. Some patients respond better to one class of NSAIDs than to another, and serial "n of 1" trials may be needed to find one that is efficacious for a given patient. NSAIDs with longer half-lives are likely to enhance compliance. NSAIDs can have significant adverse effects. Gastropathy, renal failure, and inhibition of platelet aggregation can occur with any of the nonselective medications, irrespective of the route of administration. The likelihood of these adverse effects will vary among NSAID classes and may be due, in part, to their relative COX-2 selectivity. It is important to ensure adequate hydration and good urine output in patients on NSAIDs to minimize the risk of renal vasoconstrictive injury, including papillary necrosis. Nonselective medications are relatively contraindicated in the setting of significant pre-existing renal insufficiency. NSAIDs may be contraindicated if bleeding is a problem or coagulation or platelet function is impaired. Gastric cytoprotection with misoprostol or omeprazole may be needed in patients with significant risk of gastrointestinal (GI) problems. Significant risk factors include a history of gastric ulcers or bleeding, current nausea/vomiting, protein wasting, cachexia, and advanced age.

There are parenteral forms of NSAIDs now available for use. A new transdermal form of diclofenac is now available in the United States. Its efficacy has been demonstrated in osteoarthritis[17] but has not yet been studied in localized somatic cancer pain. Ketorolac is available in intravenous (IV) or intramuscular formulations. Short-term (<5 days is considered safe in healthy patients) parenteral use of this potent agent provides excellent analgesia, particularly with visceral pain, and avoids the common central nervous system (CNS) side effects of the opioid analgesics. These advantages must be carefully weighed against the GI, renal, cardiovascular, and bleeding risks for each patient before use.

Step 2 and step 3 analgesics

Step 2 and 3 analgesics involve opioid use. The clinician must have an excellent command of opioid pharmacology when using these analgesics. Step 2 agents all have aspirin or acetaminophen present in amounts that limit their dosages to 10 to 12 tablets a day. These agents have a role in moderate pain (4–7/10), but each also has side effects. Codeine derivatives tend to be constipating, and nausea is not infrequent. There are patients who lack the necessary enzyme to convert codeine to its active (morphine) moiety. Therefore, be aware of the need to change to morphine or a step 3 agent if no analgesia is seen. Effective treatment in the ED requires a clear understanding of the pharmacology, clinical setting, and adverse effects of the analgesics prescribed and knowledge of how these may vary from patient to patient.

PRINCIPLES OF OPIOID THERAPY
Opioid Pharmacology

Opioid analgesic effect correlates with maximal plasma concentration (Cmax) (**Table 1**). Once Cmax is reached, both the maximum analgesic effect and the maximum side-effect profile have been attained. All pure opioids (except methadone) follow first-order kinetics and act in a very similar pharmacologic manner. They reach their time to peak plasma concentration (Tmax) approximately 60 to 90 minutes after oral (including enteral feeding tube) administration, 30 minutes after subcutaneous or

Table 1
Time to maximal concentration (Tmax)

Route	Time to Maximal Concentration
Intravenous	6–10 min
Rectal/subcutaneous	30 min
Oral	60–90 min

intramuscular injection or rectal administration, and 6 to 10 minutes after intravenous injection. They are eliminated from the body in a linear and predictable way, proportional to the dose. They are first conjugated in the liver, and then the kidneys excrete 90% to 95% of the metabolites. Their metabolic pathways do not become saturated. Because of its complicated cytochrome metabolism, methadone does not follow the first-order kinetics and should not be initiated or titrated in the ED without the consultation of the patient's primary care physician or a specialist in pain or palliative medicine. Each opioid metabolite has a half-life ($t\frac{1}{2}$) that depends on its rate of renal clearance. When renal function is normal, codeine, hydrocodone, hydromorphone, morphine, oxycodone, and their metabolites all have effective half-lives of approximately 3 to 4 hours. When dosed repeatedly, their plasma concentrations approach a steady state after 4 to 5 half-lives. Thus, steady-state plasma concentrations are usually attained within a day.

Opioids and their metabolites are primarily excreted renally (90%–95%). Care should be taken when dosing these agents in patients with renal impairment. The clinician should take care in selecting appropriate agents in patients with renal impairment and be prepared to reduce the dose (**Tables 2** and **3**). Morphine has 2 principal metabolites: morphine-3-glucuronide and morphine-6-glucuronide. Morphine-6-glucuronide is active and has a longer half-life than that of the parent drug morphine. Consequently, when dehydration or acute or chronic renal failure impairs renal clearance, the dosing interval for morphine must be increased or the dosage size decreased to avoid excessive accumulation of active drug and metabolites.[18–20] If urine output is minimal (oliguria) or none (anuria), routine dosing should be stopped, and morphine should be administered only as needed. This is particularly important when patients are dying. Renal excretion is somewhat less of a concern with hydromorphone, but fentanyl and methadone are considered the safest choices in renal

Table 2
Opioid selection in renal failure

Opioid	Renal Failure	Dialyzable	
		Parent Drug	Metabolites
Methadone	Appears safe	+	+
Fentanyl	Appears safe	+/−	none
Morphine	Use with caution/dose adjust	+	+
Hydromorphone		+	+/−
Hydrocodone		+	+/−
Oxycodone		Inadequate data	Inadequate data
Codeine	Do not use	Inadequate data	Inadequate data
Meperidine		Inadequate data	Inadequate data
Propoxyphene		−	−

Table 3
Opioid dose reduction in renal failure

Creatinine Clearance	Dose Reduction of Normal Dose
>50 mL/min; normal dosing	Normal
10–50 mL/min	75% dosing
<10 mL/min	50% dosing

failure. Opioid metabolism is not as sensitive to hepatic compromise. However, if hepatic function becomes severely impaired, the dosing interval should be increased or the dose decreased.

Opioid-Naïve Patients

Patients with severe pain who have never been on opioids will need a trial of short-acting opioids to establish their opioid needs and any possible respiratory depressive effect. Oral agonist opioids are appropriate for severe pain if time and circumstance allow. On an outpatient basis, severe pain may be treated with WHO step 3 analgesics as a reasonable first choice. If an immediate-release oral opioid is selected, and the pain is persistent or nearly so, the medication should be given every 4 hours. Once steady state has been reached, the best possible pain control for the dose will be achieved within a day (4–5 half-lives). The patient should see his or her primary physician within the next 24 to 48 hours, and he or she should be started on long-acting, continuous-release medications with breakthrough doses as needed.

Opioid-Tolerant Patients

Opioid-tolerant patients may come to the ED experiencing oligoanalgesia. They often say that their medications are no longer effective. This can be a function of physiologic tolerance, disease progression, or ineffective use of the medications (for example, taking continuous-release opioids only once per day when they were intended for 12-hour use). Opioid-tolerant patients presenting to the ED with severe pain will often need to have increases made in their baseline opioid dosing to achieve pain control.

RESPIRATORY DEPRESSION, NALOXONE, AND DOUBLE EFFECT

Emergency clinicians have a variety of concerns that make providing appropriate dosing of opioids challenging. Emergency staff, patients, and families often have concerns of addiction, misuse of the drug, and unintended outcomes, such as respiratory depression. The actual risk of respiratory depression is likely exaggerated due to the inappropriate application of animal and human models from acute pain research in opioid-naïve subjects. Respiratory depression is very unlikely in the treatment of cancer pain for patients with stable organ function.[21] The risks for respiratory depression include patients with advanced age, obesity, sleep apnea, impaired liver or renal function, side effect of sedation, and patients who achieve good pain control after long periods of poor pain control (**Box 1**).

Pain is a potent stimulus to breathe, and pharmacologic tolerance to respiratory depression develops quickly.[22] In similar doses, opioid effects are quite different in patients who are in pain and those who are not in pain. As doses increase, respiratory depression does not occur suddenly in the absence of other signs of overdose, such as lethargy and somnolence. In addition, somnolence always precedes respiratory depression. The presence of unusual somnolence provides an objective guide for

| **Box 1** |
| **Risk factors for respiratory depression** |

Patients at increased risk for respiratory depression

- Patients who are opioid naïve
- Patients of advanced age
- Obese patients
- Patients with sleep apnea
- Patients with impaired liver or renal function
- Patients with side effect of sedation
- Patients who achieve good pain control after long periods of poor pain control

safe downward adjustments (or the rare need for intervention) before the onset of respiratory depression. In addition, tolerance to the respiratory depressant effects of opioids occurs rapidly (a few days in most cases). Therefore, opioid-tolerant patients are much less susceptible to these effects.

Adequate ongoing assessment and appropriate titration of opioids based on pharmacologic principles will prevent misadventures. As physiologic conditions change, opioid tolerance may change. Opioid-related respiratory depression may be an indication of a physiologic change in the patient, such as worsening renal or hepatic function, ileus, or bowel obstruction. In addition, patients who develop fever or apply heat to a transdermal patch can rapidly and dangerously elevate the drug levels. In such a situation, the removal of the transdermal patch is analogous to decontamination in an acute poisoning and should be done as quickly as possible.

Naloxone may be necessary if the cause of serious respiratory depression (rate <6/min) is an opioid. If Emergency Medical Service is called to the home of a patient for unexpected respiratory depression, an important immediate goal is to avoid an acute withdrawal state. A safe method of intervening while avoiding acute withdrawal is to dilute 0.4 mg naloxone into 10 mL of normal saline (0.04 mg/mL). Administer 0.5 mL IV every 1 to 2 minutes until respirations increase but generally not to the point of alertness. Because the effective plasma half-life is short (10–15 minutes) and because of naloxone's high affinity for lipids, the patient should be closely monitored every few minutes for recurrent drowsiness. If drowsiness recurs, dosing should be repeated (occasionally a continuous infusion is needed) as required until the patient is no longer compromised.[23]

If the primary goal of care is comfort in a patient whose only conscious experience is excruciating pain, then permissive somnolence might be acceptable. In an actively dying patient, while treating the patient's suffering with appropriate dosing of medications, the patient may finally stop breathing. With the severely impaired physiology of the actively dying patient, the addition of medications to alleviate suffering consistent with the patient's goals of care might contribute to his or her death in an unknowable way. This is the principle of "double effect," which depends entirely on the intention and actions of the treating clinician. If the clinician is using accepted medical practice to treat suffering appropriately and the patient dies, the clinician's intention has been only to alleviate symptoms. If the intention were to induce death with a dose of medication that will likely result in the patient's death, then the practice would be referred to as "physician-assisted suicide." Physician-assisted suicide is illegal in the United States except in Oregon, where its practice is carefully monitored.

OPIOID DOSING STRATEGIES

In order to provide rapid, adequate, and safe pain relief with opioids in the ED, it is important to know a patient's current medication regime. Increasing dosages by 25% to 50% per day when moderate pain persists or by 50% to 100% per day for patients with continued severe pain is considered safe practice. Understanding the pharmacokinetics of opioids, it is nevertheless prudent for patients to be observed at home during the next 24 hours (until steady state is achieved) for signs of dose-limiting toxicity. The emergency clinician should always speak with the primary care outpatient provider to ensure that the opioids can be effectively titrated and the patient receives follow-up care.

Equianalgesic dosing tables help to convert a sometimes complex array of multiple medications into a single opioid equivalent (**Table 4**). From there, a safe and effective dose for initial treatment can be implemented. When converting from one opioid to another, a helpful first step is to calculate the "oral morphine equivalent" of the patient's current opioid. The oral morphine equivalent is the dose of morphine that is of equivalent strength to the dose of the current opioid. It is usually calculated for the preceding 24-hour time period. For example, a patient who is taking 4 mg of oral hydromorphone every 4 hours is receiving 24 mg of oral hydromorphone in a 24-hour period. The oral morphine equivalent of 24 mg of oral hydromorphone is approximately 90 mg of oral morphine (24 [30/7.5] = 96, rounded down to 90). This is equivalent to 30 mg IV/subcutaneous (SQ) morphine. Accepted guidelines for the conversion of transdermal fentanyl to oral morphine are unusual in that the hourly dose of the transdermal form is equated to the daily (24 h) dose of oral morphine. For example, a 25 mcg/h transdermal fentanyl patch (which is typically maintained for 3 days) is roughly equivalent to 50 mg of oral morphine a day.[24]

OPIOID CROSS-TOLERANCE

Although patients may develop pharmacologic tolerance (a higher dose to achieve the same effect) to the opioid being used, tolerance may not be as marked relative to other opioids. Incomplete cross-tolerance is likely due to subtle differences in the molecular structure of each opioid and the way each interacts with the patient's opioid receptors. Consequently, when switching opioids, there may be differences between published equianalgesic doses of different opioids and the effective dose for a given patient. It is prudent to start with 50% to 75% of the published equianalgesic dose of the new opioid to compensate for incomplete cross-tolerance and individual variation, especially if the patient's pain is controlled. If the patient has moderate to severe pain, the dose should not be reduced as much. If the patient has had adverse effects such as sedation, the dose should be reduced even more. However, in the case of

Table 4		
Equianalgesic opioid dosing table		
Equianalgesic Doses of OPIOID Analgesics		
Oral/Rectal Dose (mg)	**Analgesic**	**Parenteral Dose (mg)**
100	Codeine	60
15	Hydrocodone	—
4	Hydromorphone	1
15	Morphine	5
10	Oxycodone	—

a known time-limited side effect such as nausea, the dose may be continued with a trial of treatment of the side effect.

An important exception is methadone. Methadone is the only opioid shown to have a nonlinear relationship to standard opioids. For patients receiving morphine doses less than 100 mg/d, the ratio is 4:1 (morphine:methadone). However if the morphine is >1000 mg/d, the ratio is 20:1 (morphine:methadone).[23] Conversion to methadone is complex and requires expertise in the use of the drug. Expertise with administering methadone as well as close follow-up is essential for safety. Emergency clinicians should discuss any methadone dosing with a pain or palliative care consultant before adjustments to assist as well as ensure safe use.

BREAKTHROUGH DOSING

Treatment in cancer pain is guided by knowledge of the patient's current medications and dosing for baseline and breakthrough pain. Baseline pain refers to the patient's pain experience for more than 12 hours in a 24-hour period. Breakthrough pain is a moderate to severe transient increase over baseline pain.[25] Breakthrough dosing is typically 5% to 15% of the total daily dose in oral morphine equivalents every hour (Cmax). Any immediate-release opioid can be used, but care must be taken to avoid acetaminophen toxicity when combination medications are used for breakthrough dosing. Extended-release opioids should not be used for breakthrough pain, as their onset of action is too slow, and risk for cumulative toxicity is high.

BOLUS EFFECT

As the level of opioid in the bloodstream increases due to use of immediate-release preparations, some patients may experience drowsiness 1/2 to 1 hour after ingestion, when the plasma level peaks. This may be followed by pain just before the next dose is due, when the plasma level falls. The name of this syndrome is the "bolus effect," and it can best be resolved by switching to an extended-release formulation (oral, rectal, or transdermal) or a continuous parenteral infusion. This should reduce swings in the plasma concentration after each dose.[26]

ADJUVANT ANALGESICS

Adjuvant analgesics (or coanalgesics) are medications that, when added to primary analgesics, further improve pain control. They may themselves also be primary analgesics (eg, tricyclic antidepressant medications for postherpetic neuralgia). They can be added into the pain management plan at any step in the WHO ladder and are often used. Common adjuvants include the WHO step 1 medications as well as other medications used in the treatment of neuropathic pain.

Corticosteroids are potent anti-inflammatory agents that are useful in both nociceptive and neuropathic pain. Reducing inflammation and peritumor edema can be important in relieving pressure on a nerve or the spinal cord, decreasing intracranial pressure from a brain tumor, or decreasing obstruction of a hollow viscus. Corticosteroids may also be useful for bone pain, visceral pain (obstruction and/or capsular distention), anorexia, nausea, and depressed mood. At the end of life, dexamethasone is considered the corticosteroid of choice because of its minimal mineralocorticoid effects and thus its decreased tendency for salt and fluid retention. Corticosteroids may also enhance pain control through the creation of a sense of euphoria. Dexamethasone has a long half-life (>36 hours). It can be administered once a day in doses of 2 to 20 mg oral or up to 100 mg IV for acute spinal cord compression. If an agitated delirium ensues, steroid psychosis should be considered. Although proximal myopathy, oral candidiasis, bone loss, and other toxicities may occur with long-term use, this is seldom a major problem in the setting of advanced disease.

ROUTES OF ADMINISTRATION

The oral route is generally the least invasive and most convenient for administering opioids on a routine basis. However, some patients may benefit from other routes of administration if oral intake is either not possible (due to vomiting, dysphagia, or esophageal obstruction) or if it causes uncontrollable adverse effects (nausea, drowsiness, or confusion).

Enteral feeding tubes provide alternatives for bypassing gastroesophageal obstructions. They deliver the medications to the stomach or upper intestine where the medications function pharmacologically as though they had been ingested orally. Immediate-release medications or liquid medications are easily administered through feeding tubes. Long-acting preparations, however, cannot be crushed for administration. One long-acting morphine preparation Kadian has multiple time-release granules that may be removed from the capsule and administered through the feeding tube as a 24-hour, long-acting opioid. Transmucosal (buccal mucosal) administration of more concentrated, immediate-release, liquid preparations provides a similar alternative, particularly in the patient who is unable to swallow. Oral transmucosal fentanyl citrate is a formulation of fentanyl in a candy matrix on a stick that is approved for the treatment of breakthrough pain. To date, experience with this formulation and the recently released fentanyl dissolvable tablet show some usefulness for breakthrough pain, although dosing and cost are problematic. Topical anesthetic creams are currently used most commonly in pediatrics in the ED and are effective. They should be considered as well for cancer patients. Venipuncture may be intolerably painful to a patient in severe discomfort. If it is acceptable in a given situation to wait for a necessary venipuncture, topical analgesia with agents such as eutectic mixture of local anesthetics (lidocaine 2.5%/prilocaine 2.5%) or ELA-Max (4% lidocaine) should be considered.

Open wounds may also be a source of considerable pain, particularly during dressing changes or debridement. If incident pain is significant, the patient should be given medication before performing activities that cause pain. Based on Cmax for opioids, this could be 60 minutes for oral medications, 30 minutes for SQ or rectal, and 15 minutes for IV (see **Table 1**). It should be noted that these are the most conservative figures and that the Tmax of IV morphine is often quoted at 6 to 8 minutes.

In addition, topical analgesics should be considered. It is known that there are *mu* opioid receptors throughout the body, and there is some experience with the successful use of the IV form of morphine applied topically. This may be placed topically into the wound during a dressing change. Depending on the size of the wound and opioid tolerance of the patient, 4 to 20 mg of injectable morphine can be placed into an inert cream and applied directly to the wound and covered with gauze dressings.[27–29]

Transdermal patches present an effective alternative route of administration for patients who are receiving stable routine opioid dosing. These patches are currently manufactured only with fentanyl, and they perform quite differently from other extended-release formulations. Steady-state equilibrium is established between the medication in the patch, a subdermal pool that develops, and the patient's circulation. On average, best possible pain control is achieved within 1 dosing interval (ie, 3 days), with peak effect at about 24 hours. The effect usually lasts for 48 to 72 hours before the patch needs to be changed. Care must be taken to ensure that the patches are placed in an appropriate location so they absorb properly and adhere to the patient's skin.

Fentanyl is highly lipophilic, so an area with adequate subcutaneous fat and no hair is the best choice. It is also important to understand that if the patch needs to be removed, the drug will continue to exert an effect for up to 12 hours after removal.

Rectal administration of prepackaged suppositories or extended-release oral morphine tablets inserted rectally behave pharmacologically like related oral preparations. This route may be very effective if oral intake is suddenly not possible, although many patients do not like this route for continuous administration.

Parenteral (IV or subcutaneous) administration using injection or infusion can be very useful in some patients. If bolus dosing is required, and IV access is either not present or difficult, the subcutaneous route is an appropriate route. The intramuscular route is not recommended. Intermittent subcutaneous injections are much less painful and just as effective. When renal function is normal, routine parenteral bolus (IV or SQ) doses should be provided every 3 hours and the dose adjusted every 12 to 24 hours once steady state is reached. If a parenteral route will be used for some time, continuous infusions may produce a more constant plasma level, reduce the risk of adverse effects, be better tolerated by the patient, and require less intervention by professional staff. Patient-controlled analgesia has been shown to be both effective and well tolerated by patients. Although intravenous infusions may be preferable when intravenous access is already established and in use for other medications, all opioids available for parenteral use may be administered subcutaneously without the discomfort associated with searching for an IV site or the risk of serious infection. Either 25- or 27-gauge needles can be used for both bolus dosing and infusions. The needles can be left in place for 7 days or more as long as there is no sign of infection or local irritation. Family members can be taught to change the needles.

Pain from tumor infiltration can cause excruciating pain, which is sometimes resistant to medications. In addition, the side effects of systemic medications used to treat pain are sometimes intolerable, even with significant supportive treatment. Anesthetic techniques such as neuraxial (epidural or intrathecal) catheter delivery of pain medication or anesthetic blocks of the involved area can sometimes help dramatically. These approaches are available through specialists in interventional pain management. This is an excellent consideration for patients with pain that is unresponsive to standard aggressive medical therapy or as an adjunct to pain management when side effects are unmanageable.

NONRECOMMENDED OPIOIDS

Not all analgesics available today are recommended. Meperidine has 2 major problems that make it undesirable, and, thus, it has been removed from many hospital formularies. Its principal metabolite, normeperidine, has no analgesic properties of its own, has a longer half-life of about 6 hours, is renally excreted, and produces significant adverse effects when it accumulates, such as tremulousness, dysphoria, myoclonus, and seizures. Additionally, meperidine is poorly absorbed orally and has a short half-life of approximately 3 hours. The routine dosing of meperidine every 3 hours for analgesia leads to unavoidable accumulation of normeperidine and exposes the patient to unnecessary risk of adverse effects, particularly if renal clearance is impaired. Consequently, meperidine is not recommended for routine dosing.

Propoxyphene is also not recommended. It has a narrow therapeutic window, standard dosing is below analgesic threshold, and dose escalation is associated with accumulation of toxic metabolites.

The mixed opioid agonist-antagonists (pentazocine, butorphanol, nalbuphine, and dezocine) cannot be used in patients who might require other opioids. If used together, competition for the opioid receptors may cause a withdrawal reaction. Furthermore, agonist-antagonists are not recommended as routine analgesics, because their dosing is limited by a ceiling effect, which precludes dose escalation, and some carry a high risk of psychotomimetic adverse effects.

OPIOID-INDUCED SIDE EFFECTS

Many people confuse opioid side effects, such as urticaria/pruritis, nausea/vomiting, constipation, drowsiness, or confusion, with allergic reactions. Although 1 or more adverse effect may present on initial dosing, they can be easily managed, and in a relatively brief period of time, patients generally develop pharmacologic tolerance to all of them (except constipation). Urticaria, pruritis, and bronchospasm could be direct opioid effects or signs of allergy. These effects are usually the result of mast cell destabilization by the opioid and subsequent histamine release. Usually, the rash and pruritis can be managed by routine administration of long-acting, nonsedating oral antihistamines while opioid dosing continues (eg, fexofenadine, 60 mg twice a day; diphenhydramine, 25 mg every 6 hours, or loratadine, 10 mg daily). True anaphylaxis, although rare with opioids, should certainly be taken very seriously, and the offending opioid should be replaced with another from a different class.

Many patients who start opioids experience nausea, with or without vomiting. It is easily anticipated and treated with antiemetics and usually disappears within a few days as tolerance develops. Young women seem to be most at risk. Dopamine-blocking agents are most often effective (eg, prochlorperazine, 10 mg before opioid and every 6 hours; haloperidol, 1 mg before opioid and every 6 hours; metoclopramide, 10 mg before opioid and every 6 hours).

PROPHYLAXIS AGAINST CONSTIPATION

Constipation secondary to opioid administration is almost universal. It is primarily the result of opioid effects on the CNS, spinal cord, and myenteric plexus of gut, which, in turn, reduce gut motor activity and increase stool transit time. The colon has more time to desiccate its contents, leaving large hard stools that are difficult to pass. Other factors, such as dehydration, poor food intake, and other medications, may make the problem worse. Tolerance to constipation may develop very slowly, if at all. It requires anticipatory and ongoing management. Dietary interventions alone (eg, increase fluid and fiber) are often insufficient. Bulk-forming agents (eg, psyllium) require substantial fluid intake and are not recommended for those with advanced disease and poor mobility.

To counteract the slowing effect of opioids, the clinician should prescribe a routine stimulant laxative (eg, senna, bisacodyl, glycerine, casanthranol, etc) and escalate the dose to effect. Although detergent laxatives or "stool softeners" (eg, docusate sodium) are usually not effective by themselves, combination stimulant/softeners (eg, senna + docusate sodium) can be useful. Prokinetic agents (eg, metoclopramide) may also counteract the opioid effect. If constipation persists, some patients will benefit from the addition of an osmotic agent, such as milk of magnesia, lactulose, or sorbitol, to increase the moisture content of the stool. Many patients have difficulty tolerating the discomfort associated with osmotic agents, so they should be considered second-line therapy when prokinetics and detergent/softener laxatives are inadequate.

When standard therapies for constipation are either inadequate or the route of administration is untenable, methylnaltrexone bromide (Relistor) may be tried.

Methylnaltrexone bromide was approved in 2008 by the FDA for use in adult patients with opioid-induced constipation in advanced illness. The mechanism of action is at the gut mu receptors, where it inhibits opioid uptake. Laxation (without diminished opioid analgesia) is expected for the majority of patients within 4 hours but as early as 30 minutes, with a single dose of 0.15 mg/kg. The drug may be administered as a single subcutaneous injection every other day as needed.[30,31]

RAPID OPIOID TITRATION IN THE ED

The administration of parenteral medication in the ED, as a time-limited therapeutic trial, allows the clinician to discover what medication level a patient can safely and effectively tolerate while the patient is still in the ED. Opioid pain management in the ED can be done rapidly, safely, and effectively if analgesic principles are used. Treating the patient in the ED to establish opioid tolerance of dosing over a period of time is an important safety guard. Because maximal side effects of sleepiness, drowsiness, and respiratory depression occur at Cmax, the emergency clinician can give the patient a test dose, observe this effect, and expect a similar state in the home setting.

Oligoanalgesia in the home environment is often a reason for a patient with malignancy to seek help in the ED. The severity of pain (assessed by an appropriate pain scale) determines the approach. If the pain is assessed as severe, a rapid titration of pain medication in the ED is indicated. Adequate pain control can be achieved rapidly and safely in the ED. There are limited studies looking at rapid titration of opioids, but safety and efficacy are consistently demonstrated using standard dosing guidelines.[32–34]

If the pain is assessed as mild to moderate (<6/10), a standard history and physical examination should help determine the best intervention in the ED. The reason for oligoanalgesia may be as simple as a misunderstanding of medication dosage or interval. Communication with the primary care physician or oncologist may provide additional information to guide further interventions as well as appropriate disposition. It may make sense to provide a medication or particular dosage in the ED, by an acceptable route to the patient, to determine efficacy. By Cmax (under 90 minutes for enteral routes), if the home situation is acceptable and simple medication or dose adjustments are likely to achieve comfort, then the patient can be safely discharged with appropriate follow-up.

The following approach to the rapid treatment of cancer pain is derived from the Educating Physicians on End of Life Care-Emergency Medicine[35] curriculum:

Step 1: Assess

- Is this pain, despite its intensity, familiar in character to the patient, or is this a new pain?
- Is this likely related to the cancer or something unrelated?
- Is this progressive baseline pain (>12/24 h) or breakthrough pain?
- What medication and dosage has the patient taken for pain control in the past 24 to 48 hours? What is the response (degree of pain relief and duration of effect) to a given dose of each medication? When was the last dose?
- If severe (>7/10), initiate treatment (step 2):
- If mild to moderate pain (and when severe pain is better controlled):
  ○ Is the patient taking home medications appropriately?
  ○ Is the pain expected to be more opioid responsive (nociceptive) or less opioid responsive (neuropathic)?

- Are appropriate adjuvant therapies being used?
- Are there serious diagnostic concerns to be addressed emergently within the patient's goals of care?

Step 2: Treat

- Severe pain (>7/10): The optimal route for rapid titration of severe pain is IV (if a port or first-attempt peripheral vein is accessible) or SQ.
  - Opioid naïve: Administer parenteral morphine equivalent to 0.1 mg/kg (less if in a high-risk group).
  - Opioid tolerant: Administer 5% of the patient's total previous 24-hour parenteral morphine equivalents, minimum 0.1 mg/kg (less if patient is in a high-risk group).
- Mild to moderate pain: Consider best route and choice of medication based on assessment and goals of care.

Step 3: Reassess

- Perform pain severity assessment at Cmax (15 minutes after completion of intravenous pyelogram or intravenous piggyback dose, 30 minutes after SQ injection, 60–90 minutes after enteral route).
- Are there unwanted side effects (somnolence, confusion)?

Step 4: Achieve Adequate Pain Control

- Persistent severe pain (>7/10) without unmanageable side effects: Double the opioid dose.
- Some response but inadequate relief of pain (<50% improvement): Repeat same opioid dose.

Repeat steps 3 and 4 until pain is controlled or unwanted side effects occur, or limit further escalation.

Step 5: Determine Plan for Disposition, Discharge Instructions, and Follow-up

- Patients who cannot be reasonably controlled over a period of dose escalation and observation in the ED should be considered for hospital admission.
- The choice of a long-acting regimen depends on the patient's previous opioid use, the ability to swallow, the allergy profile, and what has been tolerated in the past. With the exception of methadone (which may have some activity in neuropathic pain), there is no commonly accepted advantage of any particular long-acting opioid. Because of its complicated dosing, methadone should not be initiated or titrated from the ED without consultation from the patient's primary care physician or a specialist in pain or palliative medicine.
- After achieving adequate pain control with the increase in long-acting opioids accompanied by appropriate breakthrough dosing, discharge instructions and follow-up with the oncologist or primary physician should be arranged.

SUMMARY

Patients and families struggling with cancer fear pain more than any other physical symptom. A basic understanding of pain assessment, opioid pharmacology, equianalgesic conversions, rationale for opioid dose escalations, and management of side effects can enhance a clinician's ability not only to effectively manage pain but also to enhance patient safety.

REFERENCES

1. van den Beuken-van Everdingen MH, de Rijke JM, Kessels AG, et al. Prevalence of pain in patients with cancer: a systematic review of the past 40 years. Ann Oncol 2007;18(9):1437–49.
2. Ventafridda VOE, Caraceni A. A retrospective study on the use of oral morphine in cancer pain. J Pain Symptom Manage 1987;2:77–82.
3. Walker VA, Hoskin PJ, Hanks GW, et al. Evaluation of WHO analgesic guidelines for cancer pain in a hospital-based palliative care unit. J Pain Symptom Manage 1988;3:145–9.
4. Goisis A, Gorini M, Ratti R, et al. Application of a WHO protocol on medical therapy for oncologic pain in an internal medicine hospital. Tumori 1989;75: 470–2.
5. Caraceni A, Martini C, Zecca E, et al. Breakthrough pain characteristics and syndromes in patients with cancer pain. An international survey. Pa Med 2004; 18:177–83.
6. Zech DF, Grond S, Lynch J, et al. Validation of World Health Organization guidelines for cancer pain relief: a 10-year prospective study. Pain 1995;63:65–76.
7. Mercadante S. Pain treatment and outcomes for patients with advanced cancer who receive follow-up care at home. Cancer 1999;85:1849–58.
8. Moryl N, Coyle N, Foley KM. Managing an acute pain crisis in a patient with advanced cancer: "this is as much of a crisis as a code". JAMA 2008;299(12): 1457–67.
9. Todd KH. Pain assessment instruments for use in the emergency department. Emerg Med Clin North Am 2005;23:285–95.
10. Ramer L, Richardson JL, Cohen MZ, et al. Multimeasure pain assessment in an ethnically diverse group of patients with cancer. J Transcult Nurs 1999;10: 94–101.
11. DeWaters T, Faut-Callahan M, McCann JJ, et al. Comparison of self-reported pain and the PAINAD scale in hospitalized cognitively impaired and intact older adults after hip fracture surgery. Orthop Nurs 2008;27(1):28–30.
12. Zwakhalen SM, hamers JP, Berger MP. The psychometric quality and clinical usefulness of three pain assessment tools for elderly people with dementia. Pain 2006;126(1–3):210–20.
13. Foley KM. Acute and chronic cancer pain syndromes. In: Doyle D, Hanks G, Cherny K, et al, editors. Oxford textbook of palliative medicine. New York: Oxford University Press; 2004. p. 298–316.
14. Bruera E, Neumann CM, Gagnon B, et al. Edmonton Regional Palliative Care Program: impact on patterns of terminal cancer care. CMAJ 1999;161(3): 290–3.
15. Breitbart W, Chochinov HM, Passik SD. Psychiatric symptoms in palliative medicine. In: Doyle D, Hanks G, Cherny K, et al, editors. Oxford textbook of palliative medicine. New York: Oxford University Press; 2004. p. 746–71.
16. Casarett D, Pickard A, Bailey FA, et al. "Do palliative consultations improve patient outcomes?". J Am Geriatr Soc 2008;56(4):593–9.
17. Bruhlmann P, Florent dV, Dreiser, et al. Short-term treatment with topical diclofenac epolamine plaster in patients with symptomatic knee osteoarthritis: pooled analysis of two randomised clinical studies. Curr Med Res Opin 2006;22(12): 2429–38.
18. Dean M. Opioids in renal failure and dialysis patients. J Pain Symptom Manage 2004;28(5):497–504.

19. Broadbent A, Khor K, Heaney A. Palliation and chronic renal failure: opioid and other palliative medications – dosage guidelines. Progr Palliat Care 2003;11(4): 183–90.

20. Murphy EJ. Acute pain management pharmacology for the patient with concurrent renal or hepatic disease. Anaesth Intensive Care 2005;33(3):311–22.

21. Estfan B, Mahmoud F, Shaheen P, et al. Respiratory function during parenteral opioid titration for cancer pain. Pa Med 2007;21(2):81–6.

22. Smith LH. Opioid safety: is your patient at risk for respiratory depression? Clin J Oncol Nurs 2007;11(2):293–6.

23. Abrams JL. Pharmacological management of cancer pain. A physician's guide to pain and symptom management in cancer patients. Baltimore (MD): The Johns Hopkins University Press; 2005. p. 197–9, 242.

24. Skaer TL. Practice guidelines for transdermal opioids in malignant pain. Drugs 2004;64(23):2629–38.

25. Portenoy RK, Hagen NA. "Breakthrough pain: definition, prevalence and characteristics". Pain Headache 1990;41:273–82.

26. Cherny N, Ripamonti C, Pereira J, , et alExpert Working Group of the European Association of Palliative Care Network. Strategies to manage the adverse effects of oral morphine: an evidence-based report. J Clin Oncol 2001;19(9):2542–54.

27. Krajnik M, Zylicz Z, Finlay I, et al. Potential uses of topical opioids in palliative care—report of 6 cases. Pain 1999;80(1–2):121–5.

28. Zeppetella G, Paul J, Ribeiro MDC. Analgesic efficacy of morphine applied topically to painful ulcers. J Pain Symptom Manage 2003;25:555–8.

29. Zeppetella G, Ribeiro MDC. Morphine in Intrasite gel applied topically to painful ulcers. J Pain Symptom Manage 2005;29:118–9.

30. Portenoy RK, Thomas J, Boatwright MLM, et al. Subcutaneous methylnaltrexone for the treatment of opioid-induced constipation in patients with advanced illness: a double-blind, randomized, parallel group, dose-ranging study. J Pain Symptom Manage 2008;35:458–68.

31. Thomas J, Karver S, Cooney GA, et al. Methylnaltrexone for opioid-induced constipation in advanced illness. N Engl J Med 2008;358:2332–43.

32. Mercadante S, Villari P, Ferrera P, et al. "Rapid titration with intravenous morphine for severe cancer pain and immediate oral conversion". Cancer 2002;95(1): 203–8.

33. Soares LGL, Martins M, Uchoa R. Intravenous fentanyl for cancer pain: a "Fast Titration" protocol for the emergency room". J Pain Symptom Manage 2003; 26(3):876–81.

34. Hagen NA, Elwood T, Ernst S. "Cancer pain emergencies: a protocol for management". J Pain Symptom Manage 1997;14(1):45–50.

35. The EPEC Project. Module 12: Malignant Pain. In: Emanuel LL, Quest TE, editors. The education in palliative and end-of-life care-emergency medicine (EPEC-EM) trainer's guide. Chicago (IL): Northwestern University; 2008.

Index

Note: Page numbers of article titles are in **boldface** type.

Hematol Oncol Clin N Am 24 (2010) 659–668
doi:10.1016/S0889-8588(10)00073-0
0889-8588/10/$ – see front matter © 2010 Elsevier Inc. All rights reserved.

hemonc.theclinics.com

Moving?

Make sure your subscription moves with you!

To notify us of your new address, find your **Clinics Account Number** (located on your mailing label above your name), and contact customer service at:

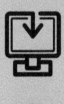

Email: journalscustomerservice-usa@elsevier.com

800-654-2452 (subscribers in the U.S. & Canada)
314-447-8871 (subscribers outside of the U.S. & Canada)

Fax number: 314-447-8029

Elsevier Health Sciences Division
Subscription Customer Service
3251 Riverport Lane
Maryland Heights, MO 63043

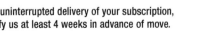

Printed and bound by CPI Group (UK) Ltd, Croydon, CR0 4YY

03/10/2024

01040444-0017